Exercise for Frail Elders

Elizabeth Best-Martini, MS CTRS
Kim A. Botenhagen-DiGenova, MA

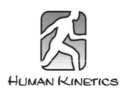

HUMAN KINETICS

Library of Congress Cataloging-in-Publication Data

Best-Martini, Elizabeth, 1948-
    Exercise for frail elders / Elizabeth Best-Martini, Kim A.
Botenhagen-DiGenova.
        p. cm.
Includes bibliographical references and index.
    ISBN 0-7360-3687-3 (softcover : alk. paper)
  1. Exercise for the aged. 2. Frail elderly--Diseases--Exercise
therapy. I. Botenhagen-DiGenova, Kim A., 1957- . II. Title.
  RC953.8.E93 B377 2003
  613.7'0446--dc21

2002151517

ISBN 0-7360-3687-3

Exercise and health are matters that vary from individual to individual. Readers should speak with their own doctors about their individual needs before starting any exercise program. This book is not intended as a substitute for the medical advice and supervision of your personal physician. Any application of the recommendations set forth in the following pages is at the reader's discretion and sole risk.

Acquisitions Editor: Judy Patterson Wright, PhD; **Developmental Editors:** Jennifer L. Walker and Melissa Feld; **Assistant Editors:** Sandra Merz Bott, Susan C. Hagan, and Derek Campbell; **Copyeditor:** Karen Bojda; **Proofreader:** Pamela Johnson; **Indexer:** Wyman Indexing/L. Pilar Wyman; **Permission Manager:** Dalene Reeder; **Graphic Designer:** Nancy Rasmus; **Graphic Artist:** Dawn Sills; **Photo Manager:** Leslie A. Woodrum; **Cover Designer:** Keith Blomberg; **Photographer (cover):** Leslie A. Woodrum; **Photographer (interior):** Leslie A. Woodrum; **Art Manager:** Kelly Hendren; **Illustrators:** Kelly Hendren and Mic Greenberg; **Printer:** United Graphics

Printed in the United States of America   10 9 8 7 6 5 4 3 2

Human Kinetics
Web site: www.HumanKinetics.com

United States: Human Kinetics
P.O. Box 5076
Champaign, IL 61825-5076
800-747-4457
e-mail: humank@hkusa.com

Canada: Human Kinetics
475 Devonshire Road, Unit 100
Windsor, ON N8Y 2L5
800-465-7301 (in Canada only)
e-mail: orders@hkcanada.com

Europe: Human Kinetics
107 Bradford Road
Stanningley
Leeds LS28 6AT, United Kingdom
+44 (0)113 255 5665
e-mail: hk@hkeurope.com

Australia: Human Kinetics
57A Price Avenue
Lower Mitcham, South Australia 5062
08 8277 1555
e-mail: liaw@hkaustralia.com

New Zealand: Human Kinetics
Division of Sports Distributors NZ Ltd.
P.O. Box 300 226 Albany
North Shore City, Auckland
0064 9 448 1207
e-mail: blairc@hknewz.com

To my dearest husband, John A. Martini, whose love for me and recognition of the importance of my work have been immeasurable gifts. Thank you from the bottom of my heart. In addition, thanks for your *hands-on* assistance with editing, photography, designing graphics and forms, and overall being a strong part of this book-writing journey.

To my "one of a kind" mom, Peggy. Your smiling face and enthusiasm while lifting weights are treasures to me. Doris, my mother-in-law, you inspire me with your energy, support, and active lifestyle.

A special dedication goes to all the elderly people who have touched my life and work. You are at the heart of this book.

Betsy Best-Martini

To my Auntie Mary, who, at 87 years of age, regularly plays tennis, walks along San Francisco's Ocean Beach, lifts weights, and goes line dancing every Monday. And to my remarkable father and stepmother, Alfred and Lois Botenhagen, who continue to live active, independent lives in their 80s. We hope that this book will help many to experience such dynamic lives as theirs.

Kim Botenhagen-DiGenova

CONTENTS

APPENDIXES

PREFACE

The concept for this book, *Exercise for Frail Elders,* originated from our relationships with elderly participants in our exercise classes. They mentored us and thus showed us the profound impact that physical activity has in each of our lives—regardless of age or situation. Today's fitness leader needs an understanding of the limitations and special needs of those with illnesses, disabilities, chronic disorders, and sedentary lifestyles. There is a direct link between losing function and losing independence. Some of the simple movements and tasks that we take for granted can slip away through inactivity. No matter how out of shape, any individual can improve his or her fitness and function through proper exercise.

The need for qualified fitness leaders increases with the growing population of older adults. This is an exciting field in which to work. You can see the benefits of your exercise program in your participants' increased function and independence.

Exercise for Frail Elders is a training manual for old and new fitness professionals. Professionals in this field include activity directors, recreation directors, wellness program directors, recreation therapists, occupational therapists, physical therapists, dance therapists, physical education teachers, adaptive physical education specialists, exercise physiologists, personal trainers, certified and noncertified fitness instructors, aerobics instructors, gerontologists, adult education instructors, college instructors, and students in specialties related to older adults. Whether you are an experienced or a beginning fitness instructor, or one who is required to follow federal or state regulations for physical exercise instruction, you will find this book to be of great value as a manual that takes you through every step of the process in teaching safe and effective exercise.

This book also stands out from other exercise books for older adults in its thorough and user-friendly presentation of special needs, including Alzheimer's disease and related dementias, arthritis, cerebrovascular accident, chronic obstructive pulmonary disease, coronary artery disease, de-pression, diabetes, hip fracture or replacement and knee replacement, hypertension, multiple sclerosis, osteoporosis, Parkinson's disease, sensory losses, and traumatic head injury. This book will prepare you to meet the challenge of instructing adults with one or more special needs.

Exercise for Frail Elders gives you the tools to plan and implement a successful exercise program. Part I, "Planning a Successful Exercise Program for Frail Elders and Adults With Special Needs," covers the participants, the exercise program, and the leader. In chapter 1 you will learn about participants' individual and special needs. In chapter 2 you will learn about the exercise program and how you can make it motivating, safe, and effective. Chapter 3 walks you through steps and strategies to be a successful leader. Part II, "Implementing an Exercise Program for Frail Elders and Adults With Special Needs," provides warm-ups, aerobics (by Janie Clark, MA, president of the American Senior Fitness Association), resistance training, and cool-down exercises (stretching and relaxation) in chapters 4 through 7, respectively. Each exercise component in chapters 4 through 7 has an easy-reference chart and photographs of the exercises. Each chapter also includes safety precautions, guidelines, seated and standing exercises, and variations and progression for the exercises.

Start with the basic seated exercises, which all of your participants can learn. Carefully progress to the basic standing exercises with participants who are able to stand safely. The seated and standing exercises are designed to be taught at the same time, which allows you to accommodate individuals with a wide variety of special needs.

In chapter 8 you will learn about putting it all together to implement an exercise program that incorporates the warm-up, aerobic, resistance, and cool-down exercises from chapters 4 through 7. You will also learn how to design, schedule, modify, progress, maintain, and monitor a fitness program for frail elders and adults with special needs.

In the back of the book are appendixes that provide you with necessary and useful forms, educational handouts, and other information to help make your role as fitness leader easier, references and suggested resources to enhance your knowledge base, and an index to enable you to find the information that you are looking for quickly.

It is our sincere hope that this book will enhance your competence and confidence in meeting the special needs of individuals in your exercise classes.

ACKNOWLEDGMENTS

Thank you to the residents of Long Life Living Residential Home who exercised with our routine twice weekly, participated in our photo shoots, and named some of the exercises. Special thanks to their wonderful instructors, Melissa Calhoun Pankowski and Connie Hirschmugl, who worked closely with us in implementing and refining the exercise program. Thanks also to Faye Chang, administrator and owner of this beautiful residential setting, who so strongly supports this program and appreciates its importance in enhancing quality of life and independence.

Thank you to the members of the Millennium Movers exercise class at Hillside Convalescent Care Center. You taught us about resiliency, determination, and fun with "attitude."

Thanks to our models (in alphabetical order) from the

College of Marin—Bill Anderson ("The Duke"), Marian Housley, John Jones, Goonja Kim, Sally Sparrowhawk, Ann Wilson, and Lucian Wernick

Long Life Living Residential Home—Nancy Barnes, True Blackburn, Marna Griffin, Josephine Murray, Catherine Power, Vicky Rivers, Lina Scherini, and Ann Steiger

Hillside Care Center—Joyce Sellers, Juliet Smith, and Jesse Tarpley

Parnow Friendship House—Ali Rostambeik

Many individuals helped us bring this book to life. We thank each of you for your contributions: the Marin Commission on Aging Strength Training Task Force, Liz Rottger in particular, who introduced the authors to one another; the Marin Association of Senior Strength Trainers (MASST) for their enthusiastic support of our book; Sandy Roberts, Director of Community Education and Services, who continually supports our College of Marin classes; the Newcombs and Ellen Roberts, who helped us in the initial stage of this project; Janie Clark, MA, for writing chapter 5 and for editing part II; (in alphabetical order) Tom Beck, Bryan A. Duff, DC; Randy Gibson, MA, MS, Lac; Jacqui Gillis, PT; Vicki Jackson, MLS; John Jones; Jon Kakleas, DC, PT; Mary Lockett, PT; Shay McKelvey, RN, MS; Stephen P. Mongiello, PT; Rev. Nano Nathan; Nicolas T. Roth, PT; Mary Dale Scheller, MSW; Robert Teasdale, MD; and Lucian Wernick, MA, for helping to create and fine-tune the exercise protocols and other valuable contributions; and Kelly Philpott Brisbois, a lawyer, elder advocate, and former fitness leader in skilled nursing in Marin County, who reviewed our medical clearance forms.

Many thanks to Judy Patterson Wright, our acquisitions editor and coach; Melissa Feld and Jennifer L. Walker, our developmental editors; Sandra Merz Bott and Karen Bojda, our copyeditors; Susan Hagan and Derek Campbell, our assistant editors; Pamela Johnson, our proofreader; Dawn Sills, our graphic artist; and Les Woodrum for his artistic photography. We appreciate your guidance and commitment to excellence.

On a personal note of acknowledgment, we thank one another for the time, dedication, friendship, and focus on fun during the past few years of walking, talking, bicycling, and swimming while "working on *the* book." Here is to more fun and fitness ahead.

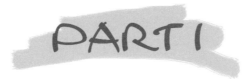

PART I

PLANNING A SUCCESSFUL EXERCISE PROGRAM FOR FRAIL ELDERS AND ADULTS WITH SPECIAL NEEDS

In chapters 1 through 3, you will learn about the participants in your exercise program, the exercise program itself, and the leader of the program. The first part of this book covers general characteristics and guidelines for these three important areas. To this framework you will add the program specifics in part II.

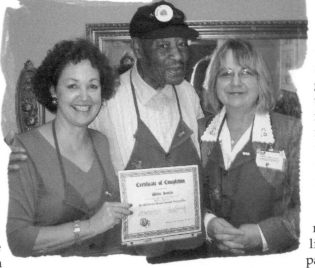

Part I is designed to help you plan a successful exercise program. Each chapter offers you easy-to-use forms, reference charts, charts of special needs, and much more. These resources help you to plan a safe and effective program that meets the needs of your participants.

Chapters 1 through 3 cover the following topics:

- Special needs of elderly participants
- Assessing the needs of individual participants
- Setting realistic goals with each participant
- Programming guidelines to increase motivation, safety, and effectiveness
- Leadership strategies and observational skills
- Group dynamics and group development

Chapter 1 introduces you to frail elders and adults with special needs. Addressing the needs of this audience is what makes this book unique. Each class is as diverse as the participants. The more you understand about medical disorders and how they affect your participants' lives and independence,

the more successful your exercise class will be. The charts in this chapter identify characteristics of people with some common medical disorders and give you easy-to-use exercise and safety tips.

Chapter 2 explains ways to make the exercise program motivating, safe, and effective. Your initial goal as the fitness leader is to keep participants coming to class and becoming more physically active, so we start by addressing motivation. The focus then moves from motivation to safety issues, including medical clearance, assessments, and safety guidelines. Responding to a participant's pain and ensuring safety while teaching a large group are both addressed. The emphasis then moves to effectiveness. Careful attention to program components helps the fitness leader design a motivating, safe, and effective program.

Chapter 3 is about you, the fitness leader, and the leadership and instructional strategies you can use to lead a fun, safe, and effective program. We start by addressing the social environment and mood of the class and some typical group goals. The next sections of the chapter take you through opening, leading, and closing the exercise class. Included in this chapter are successful strategies for teaching participants who are experiencing communication, cognitive, and sensory losses. The finishing touches of the exercise class, beyond leading the class, include your feedback to participants and all aspects of organizing supplies and space.

THE PARTICIPANTS: KNOW THEIR INDIVIDUAL NEEDS

The most important factor in teaching exercise to frail elders and adults with special needs is knowing your audience. Each group is as varied as the entire population of older adults. No generic definitions apply. You must know each person's strengths and limitations. With this information, you can tailor exercise to an individual participant and to the group as a whole.

This chapter is designed to help you better understand and recognize frailty and special needs. The primary focus is working safely and effectively with both frail elders and adults who have special needs. To meet this challenge, you need to understand common medical disorders and their implications. This chapter covers specific diagnostic areas that are relevant for frail elders and adults with special needs. With an understanding of these medical issues, you will be prepared to do the following:

- Teach exercise to participants with diverse medical needs.
- Recommend safe exercise techniques for individual participants according to their medical conditions.

Before we identify specific diagnostic areas and their implications for exercise, let's start with an examination of the terms *frail* and *special needs.*

DEFINING FRAIL ELDERS AND SPECIAL NEEDS

What age is "old" to you? We each answer this question according to our own experience with family members and with older people and how we see ourselves physically. In past years, "old" was defined by chronological age. Chronological age used to be more relevant because life expectancies were far shorter than they are today. A man of 40 in the 1800s may have been considered old. Today, an 80-year-old man may water-ski and be very physically active.

Many of us will probably live into our 70s, 80s, 90s, or 100s. In the year 2000, an estimated 35 million people—13 percent of the population—were age 65 or older. By 2030, 20 percent of Americans—about 70 million people—will have passed their 65th birthday. The fastest growing segment of the older population is people aged 85 and older (National Institute on Aging 2000).

Have you ever heard the term *old-old?* This term was created to differentiate between younger and older old people. We need this distinction because people are living so much longer. If a 65-year-old is old, then what should we call an 80-year-old? Old-old refers to the older segment of the older generation.

Of greatest importance is how we *feel* at an older chronological age and how well we can *function* physically, mentally, and emotionally. This functional status is what maintains wellness and a good quality of life. The director general of the World Health Organization refers to this as "health expectancy," as opposed to "life expectancy."

Function is a major determinant of aging successfully. As physical function declines, an individual can begin to become frail. Let's look more closely at the term *frail.*

DEFINING FRAILTY

Frail is a term that can describe anyone, young or old. *Frailty* refers to a loss of some physical function along with a possible chronic disorder and or disability. The causes of frailty vary among individuals. These are some common causes of frailty:

- A medical condition
- A loss of one or more senses
- A chronic disorder
- A chronic disorder along with a new medical diagnosis
- Changes in the musculoskeletal system
- *Sarcopenia* (loss of muscle mass)
- Very old age
- Physical inactivity

Frailty is normally due to a combination of circumstances that leave an individual unable to accomplish normal activities of daily living independently. Some people in your exercise group who are quite elderly may appear physically frail but are not. Looks can be deceiving. Function is what determines level of frailty. The possibility that you may misidentify an elderly person who is not frail as frail creates the challenge in leading exercise programs for older adults.

The term *frail elders* combines the ideas of advanced age and frailty. Normally, frail elders refers to very old people who have difficulties performing activities of daily living without assistance from others. There are added complexities to this term. An individual with a chronic disorder such as arthritis might be considered frail because of another complicating factor, such as emphysema. The combined limitations from the two disorders may contribute to the frail condition.

It is important for you to know that not all frailty is chronic or long term. Some people find themselves in a frail state caused by surgery or illness. When they recover, the frailty may decrease or disappear.

It is also possible to decrease frailty by increasing physical activity. Research has verified that exercise improves muscle strength, balance, coordination, and cardiovascular fitness in even the most frail and elderly participants. Resistance training in particular has proven to be especially beneficial with *deconditioned* (not in strong or good physical condition caused by a sedentary lifestyle) elderly individuals. Skeletal muscle weakness places an individual at higher risk of falls. These falls can lead to fractured bones and hospitalization. Strengthening and stretching exercises help maintain balance and range of motion and are recommended in many fall-prevention studies.

A report of the U.S. Surgeon General (1996), *Physical Activity and Health*, states that even moderate exercise can help frail individuals recapture lost function, functional independence, health, and well-being. This is why your exercise class is so profoundly important to this group.

DEFINING SPECIAL NEEDS

Anyone, young or old, can have special needs. A special need can be temporary or permanent. The term *special* indicates that the fitness leader needs to know what an individual's disorder or limitation is before initiating an exercise program for that individual. This large category of special needs includes a vast array of individual needs from a variety of causes.

Some special needs are related to

- a medical disorder,
- sensory losses (vision loss, loss of hearing, loss of touch),
- communication difficulties (including *aphasia* [the loss of or decline in the ability to speak, understand, read, or write] and *language barriers* [not speaking the language of the predominant culture]),
- cognitive losses,
- a sedentary lifestyle, or
- sarcopenia.

A special need may be for

- specific medical equipment (e.g., oxygen, IV),
- emotional support caused by mental health issues (e.g., depression),
- specific medications,
- adaptive equipment, or
- physical assistance with movement.

A participant may have one or more special needs that, when combined, create a frail state. For example, a participant in your group may be frail because of her age of 98 years and her poor overall physical condition. Seated next to her may be a man in his 60s with special needs related to a diagnosis of Parkinson's disease. He is an older adult with special needs, but he is 30 years younger than the frail 98-year-old. You could not call this man frail, even though he has some special needs. Seated next to these two individuals may be a younger woman who is frail and has special needs, both related to a diagnosis of multiple sclerosis. Figure 1.1 helps visually distinguish these conditions and individual needs.

COMMON MEDICAL DISORDERS IN THE ELDERLY

Some of the common medical disorders that contribute to frailty are listed in table 1.1. This section describes some of these disorders. In addition, a table for each disorder gives characteristics related to the disorder and identifies relevant safety and exercise tips (see tables 1.2 through 1.15). The tables and descriptions are intended to be a brief review. We encourage you to do further research on your own.

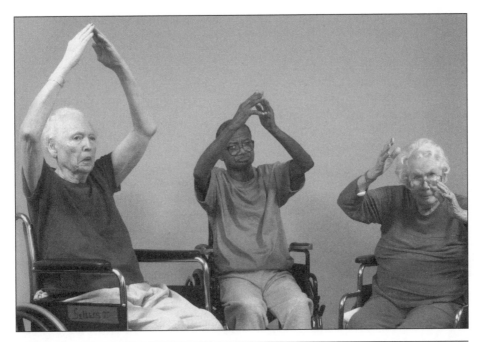

FIGURE 1.1   These three participants capture the terms *frail* and *special needs* because of advanced age, mobility issues, declining physical function, Parkinson's disease, diabetes, hypertension, cancer, and cardiac issues.

TABLE 1.1	COMMON MEDICAL DISORDERS THAT CONTRIBUTE TO FRAILTY IN ELDERLY INDIVIDUALS
System	**Medical disorder**
Cardiovascular	Hypertension, hypotension, coronary artery disease, valvular heart disease, heart failure, dysrhythmia, peripheral arterial disease
Pulmonary	Chronic obstructive pulmonary disease, pneumonia
Musculoskeletal	Arthritis, degenerative disk disease, polymyalgia rheumatica, osteoporosis, degenerative joint disease
Metabolic/endocrine	Diabetes, hypercholesterolemia
Gastrointestinal	Dental disorders, malnutrition, incontinence, diarrhea
Genitourinary	Urinary tract infection, cancer
Hematologic/immunologic	Anemia, leukemia, cancer
Neurologic	Dementia, Alzheimer's disease, cerebrovascular disease, Parkinson's disease, multiple sclerosis
Eye and ear	Cataracts, glaucoma, hearing disorders
Psychiatric	Anxiety disorders, hypochondria, depression, alcohol abuse

From *Exercise for Frail Elders* by E. Best-Martini and K.A. Botenhagen-DiGenova, 2003, Champaign, IL: Human Kinetics. Adapted, by permission, from American College of Sport Medicine, 1997, *ACSM's exercise management for persons with chronic diseases and disabilities* (Champaign, IL: Human Kinetics), 114.

ALZHEIMER'S DISEASE AND RELATED DEMENTIAS

Dementia is a neurologic disorder that is progressive and degenerative. The common definition of dementia is the progressive loss of intellectual functioning. Dementia is not a disease itself but a cluster of symptoms. *Alzheimer's disease* is one of the largest classifications of dementia. The disease begins with signs and symptoms of memory loss that begin to increase and worsen. In addition to memory loss, an individual with Alzheimer's disease experiences anxiety, as he or she loses the ability to function independently in day-to-day life. Depression is prevalent as the losses become more profound. The combination of these psychological difficulties, compounded by the inability to express oneself or understand others, is often the reason for problematic behaviors associated with dementia. Some common behaviors you may see are restlessness, wandering, crying, aggression, or withdrawal. Always communicate clearly, patiently, and compassionately with individuals who have Alzheimer's disease. Try to look beyond the behaviors and limitations and more at the person.

Other dementias are related to traumatic brain damage, cerebrovascular accidents (strokes), AIDS, Parkinson's disease, and substance abuse. The most important fact to remember about dementia is that it is a brain injury. The symptoms and behaviors are all related to the injury. The person still remains. Even people with advanced dementia retain strengths and abilities. Regardless of the level of dementia, these individuals feel the respect and care that they receive from others emotionally if not intellectually.

Although individuals with dementia struggle with intellectual functions, they usually are ambulatory (in the early and middle stages of the disease) and can be interested in physical activity. This is a strength that they still retain. Physical exercise is vitally important to their well-being; it helps maintain their physical functioning as long as possible.

Because many individuals with dementia are in good physical condition, you should focus on their strengths rather than their limitations. This enhances their self-esteem. In an exercise class, participants with dementia may have difficulty staying focused and following directions. The leadership skills for working with participants with cognitive losses are discussed in chapter 3.

TABLE 1.2	SPECIAL NEEDS OF PARTICIPANTS WITH ALZHEIMER'S DISEASE AND RELATED DEMENTIA DISORDERS
Characteristic	**Exercise and safety tips**
Memory loss	Do not anticipate carryover skills from one class to the next. Use exercises that enhance current skills.
Short attention span	Repetition helps learning and retention. Repeat directions both verbally and visually. Counting or clapping with the exercises increases attention.
Overreaction	Keep your voice and demeanor calm and reassuring. Avoid trying to explain the situation. Instead, distract and reassure.
Misunderstanding	Avoid over-stimulating this participant. Give easy directions and positive responses. Too much music or noise and too many directions and distractions can increase anxiety. Keep it simple.
Difficulty communicating	Always make eye contact. Rely on body language more than spoken words. Listen for the meaning behind the words. Use clear and simple language. Ask simple questions that require a yes or no answer. When you get to know the individual better, you can use a more individualized communication style. Introduce an exercise one step at a time with visual and verbal cues.

Characteristic	Exercise and safety tips
Anxiety and depression	Focus on the abilities and strengths that the participant still has intact. Help the participant build on what he or she does well.
	If the participant feels that you are genuine and friendly, he or she will respond at a higher level.
	Physical activity helps alleviate restlessness and anxiety.
Spatial or perceptual problems	Keep the environment uncluttered because depth perception and ability to judge distances are altered with this disease.
	Use brightly colored supplies and workout attire. Colorful ribbons, scarves, balls, balloons, parachute games, and Velcro catch games elicit a greater response from this audience.
Apraxia (inability to purposefully move the body in relationship to the environment)	Mobility is extremely important for functional stability. Use exercises based on everyday movements, such as "sweeping the floor," "reaching," "dancing," etc. These activities tap into long-term memory, which is still intact for many people with dementia.
Need for visual and tactile cues	Participants with dementia respond well to physical prompts (e.g., hand-over-hand experiences) and to touch. Remember to ask permission before touching them.
Balance problems (due to decreased postural reflexes)	Muscular strength reduces the risk of falling.

ARTHRITIS

Arthritis is a general term that refers to many rheumatic diseases that cause pain, stiffness, and swelling in joints and connective tissues (National Institutes of Health, Arthritis and Musculoskeletal and Skin Diseases 2001). The most common types of arthritis are osteoarthritis and rheumatoid arthritis. Many of the symptoms of these two types of arthritis are similar. A less common type of arthritis is fibromyalgia.

Osteoarthritis is characterized by joint pain. The pain is due to the breakdown of the *articular cartilage* (tissue that covers and protects the end of the bones). Without this cartilage, the bone edges become rough and do not move smoothly on one another. In addition, bone spurs (osteophytes) may develop. Osteoarthritis does not always cause the symptom of inflammation.

Rheumatoid arthritis is an inflammatory, multijoint, multisystem disease. It is defined as an *autoimmune disorder* (an immune or allergic reaction of the body against itself) because it affects not only the lining of the joint, but also other organs and systems (the cardiac and pulmonary systems). Swelling, along with pain and stiffness, occurs with rheumatoid arthritis. Rheumatoid arthritis causes acute episodes of joint pain and inflammation. The duration of these flare-ups varies. There may be periods of few or no flare-ups, referred to as remissions. Participants with rheumatoid arthritis have a greater tendency toward fatigue. Because of this, remind them to pace themselves and go slowly.

Fibromyalgia is a chronic pain in the soft tissue (ligaments and tendons) and muscles surrounding the joints. The pain is often experienced in the shoulder and hip regions. Treatment for this disorder is multidisciplinary and utilizes physical therapy, relaxation techniques, and lifestyle changes to eliminate the triggers (such as stress, inactivity, lack of sleep, etc.). One of the most important components of treatment for fibromyalgia is a safe exercise program.

CEREBROVASCULAR ACCIDENT (STROKE)

A *cerebrovascular accident* (CVA), or stroke, is a circulatory accident that results in neurologic impairment. It occurs when blood flow to the brain is interrupted. This can occur in two ways.

1. *Ischemic stroke* occurs when an artery is blocked and no blood can get through to a portion of the brain. There are two different types of ischemic strokes. One is caused by a fixed blood clot, or thrombosis. The other is caused by a wandering blood clot, or embolism. Ischemic stroke is the most common type of stroke. Both of these strokes occur because of a buildup of fatty deposits, referred to as *atherosclerotic plaques*, in the blood vessels of the neck and head. A stroke is sometimes referred to as

TABLE 1.3	SPECIAL NEEDS OF PARTICIPANTS WITH ARTHRITIS
Characteristic	**Exercise and safety tips**
Joint pain	Avoid fatiguing muscles, as this can increase joint pain.
	Mild isometric exercises can help to build up the muscles and decrease stress on the joints. However, this type of exercise should be offered only with the physician's approval as it increases blood pressure. We recommend that isometrics be done only individually, not in a group.
	Remind participants to take their oral pain relievers about one hour before exercising.
	Any exercise that causes joint pain that lasts longer than two hours after the exercise class should be modified or replaced with another exercise.
	Remind participants to place a pillow under an affected joint when they are relaxing at home. This helps to decrease joint pain.
Joint strain and joint instability	By decreasing body weight, a participant can reduce strain on the joints.
	Avoid positions that can lead to joint deformity (e.g., gripping a dumbbell or side bar too tightly for an extended amount of time).
	Participants with arthritis should avoid overstretching, which can damage the supportive ligaments.
Stiffness	Always warm up slowly to avoid exercise when the joints are cold and stiff.
	Participants should try not to keep the joints in the same position for too long, which can make it difficult to straighten them out fully without pain.
Decreased range of motion	Remind participants to move through only a pain-free range of motion. Participants should stay below their pain threshold.
	If participants experience any pain, they should stop exercising.
	Range-of-motion exercises before bed can decrease stiffness in the morning.
Limited endurance and fatigue	Short and frequent exercise sessions are better tolerated.
	Vary the aerobics and resistance training on different days of the week.
	Try leading exercise at different times of the day. Different people feel more flexible and more energetic at different times of the day. Endurance takes time to build. Each participant should go at his or her own pace.
Muscle weakness	Allow short pauses during exercise to help prevent joint inflammation.
	Exercise can strengthen the joints and supporting muscles, tendons, and ligaments.
Acute pain episodes in rheumatoid arthritis	During acute episodes, avoid exercising the affected joint.
	Range-of-motion exercises are recommended *if possible* during an acute stage.
	Some participants with rheumatoid arthritis may never be able to tolerate resistance training. However, body-weight exercises (see chapter 6) may be indicated.
Low energy and mood	Exercising can uplift mood and help decrease depression.
	Exercise also increases energy, which counteracts depression and anxiety.
Lower-back pain	Many people with osteoarthritis or fibromyalgia experience lower-back pain. Encourage slow movements and back exercises that are recommended by their physicians or physical therapists.
	It is important for participants to avoid becoming deconditioned, which can exacerbate back pain. Encourage participants to exercise safely through a pain-free range of motion.
Poor postural stability	Teach posture exercises to enhance joint function during exercising.
	Poor posture and awkward body movements affect walking gait, increase potential for falls, and more readily tire a participant. Proper exercise combats these negative effects.

TABLE 1.4	SPECIAL NEEDS OF PARTICIPANTS AFTER CEREBROVASCULAR ACCIDENT (STROKE)
Characteristic	**Exercise and safety tips**
Possible paralysis (hemiplegia) or weakness (hemiparesis) on one side of the body	Encourage the participant to work the affected side by having the strong arm help move the affected arm or leg in exercises. Be aware of participants' positioning in the chair during seated exercises, as they may not be able to feel whether they are sitting safely. Remind the participant to keep the affected arm on the lap for protection and avoid letting it hang over the side of the chair.
Drop foot	Make sure the participant is aware of foot placement (under chair or table) to avoid injury.
Loss of sensation or weakness	Participant may not feel heat, cold, or pain if the affected hand or foot is in an unsafe position. Encourage participant to visually check placement of the affected hand or foot for safety awareness.
Lability (inability to control inappropriate laughing or crying)	Acknowledge emotional responses and remind participants that they experience these responses as a result of the stroke. Encourage deep breathing to relax and refocus (see chapters 4 and 7).
Difficulty with new learning	Review a movement with verbal (oral) cues along with demonstration rather than having it written visually on a board, to enhance these participants' learning. Give participants extra time to respond to new movements, as they may be cautious about trying new things and have a delayed response to new information.
Posture awareness	Encourage participants to focus on their posture while sitting in a chair. They should sit all the way back in the chair. If they fall to one side or their affected arm hangs over the side of the chair, verbally remind them to reposition. Have them use the strong hand to pick up the affected arm and place it in their lap. Use exercises that involve both sides of the body. They enhance balance and coordination. Exercise movements that take the participant off the midline or center of balance help build balance control. Some exercise ideas are ball tossing or kicking. Trying to catch a ball on the neglected side enhances both balance and body awareness. Avoid any position that significantly lowers the head, such as touching toes. This may cause undue pressure within the brain.
Communication deficits, including expressive aphasia (inability to express oneself), receptive aphasia (inability to receive information clearly), or global aphasia (both)	Make directions simple, and visually demonstrate them. Give participants positive feedback on their performance.
Spasticity (increased muscle tone, stiff muscles that resist passive stretching) or flaccidity (decreased muscle tone, limp muscles)	Exercises to restore mobility and normalize the muscle tone are recommended. When the arm is flaccid, there is a greater risk of shoulder injury due to subluxation (separation of the joint surfaces). A lap board, foam wedge, or pillow can be placed on the lap or chair to support the arm while sitting and thus keep it from hanging and becoming edemic (swollen). This also protects the shoulder area. Be cautious about overhead exercises that could exacerbate the subluxation.

a brain attack because of its similarity to a heart attack, which is due to atherosclerotic plaque buildup in the coronary arteries of the heart (Gordon 1993).

2. *Hemorrhagic stroke* occurs when an artery leading to the brain ruptures. This rupture, known as a cerebral hemorrhage, spills blood into the brain or a surrounding area between the outer surface of the brain and the skull. In some instances, a congenital weak spot called an aneurysm may cause this type of stroke.

A stroke affects the area of the brain where the blood flow ceased (ischemic) or from the intracranial pressure created from the ruptured blood vessel. In addition, it may cause pressure to the brain that may result in swelling. Depending on the location of the stroke and the extent of the damage to brain tissue, stroke victims' symptoms and limitations vary. If the right side of the brain is affected, the left side of the body exhibits weakness or paralysis, or vice versa.

Here are some problems specific to the location of a CVA:

Right-side CVA	**Left-side CVA**
Spatial or perceptual problems	Speech and language deficits
Memory deficits	Memory deficits
Impulsive behavior and overestimated abilities	Difficulty with new tasks
Left field of vision restricted	Right field of vision restricted
Unawareness (neglect) of left side of body	Problems knowing left from right
Weakness or paralysis on left side	Weakness or paralysis on right side

Commonly, the most significant benefits of rehabilitation and exercise can be achieved in the first two years from the time of the initial stroke. Individuals differ in their injuries and rehabilitation; there is no specific timeline as many individuals will experience some level of functional improvement with continued exercises after this initial two-year period. We do know that exercise enhances circulation, builds up endurance, and strengthens the body. All of these contribute to better quality of life and support recovery to the greatest extent.

The first week after a stroke is the most crucial in determining its extent, severity, and potential recovery. During this time, the medical team analyzes and assesses what damage has occurred. The reha-

bilitation and exercise aspects of stroke recovery begin immediately after this assessment has been made. Many stroke victims' recovery is slow, and their prognoses for complete recovery guarded. Regardless of the prognosis for a full recovery, range-of-motion movements and basic motor skill progression are extremely important. In addition, aerobic exercise is important in keeping the fatty deposits from building up again in the blood vessels. Participants in an exercise class who have had a CVA should be discouraged from any fast movements of the head and neck. Remind them to move slowly through the exercises.

CHRONIC OBSTRUCTIVE PULMONARY DISEASE

Chronic obstructive pulmonary disease (COPD) is a category of pulmonary disorders that includes emphysema, chronic bronchitis, and asthma. In each of these disorders, the lungs are inefficient or ventilation (the passage of air into and out of the respiratory tract) is compromised. Many people may have only one type of COPD. Others may have a combination of several types if the initial disorder was not diagnosed for a long time and progressed to further lung damage.

Smokers are at higher risk of developing COPD (which is the fourth leading cause of death in the United States and affects the lives of 30 million Americans). COPD can also be caused working or living in an environment with toxins that damage the lungs. Asthma can sometimes be reversed if it originated from environmental triggers. If reversal is not possible, avoiding the environmental triggers may lessen asthmatic symptoms.

COPD does not occur overnight. It is gradual and progressive. Because ventilation is compromised, an individual with COPD finds himself or herself breathing ineffectively, wheezing, coughing, and gasping for air. This difficulty breathing is called *dyspnea*.

Breaths may be short, shallow, and too rapid to successfully provide the needed level of oxygen. Because of this lack of oxygen, physical endurance and stamina are seriously compromised. Dyspnea worsens if an individual becomes fearful of physical activity.

In addition to difficulty breathing, many individuals experience frequent periods of anxiety. Not being able to breathe can be an extremely stressful experience. A person with COPD may avoid situations that cause an emotional response such as laughing or crying. Laughing and crying both place additional demands on the already compromised breathing function. Individuals with COPD do not normally feel comfortable in small spaces or large groups. They need to pay attention to any toxins that might exacerbate their condition. Lifestyle changes associated with COPD may also cause depression. Approximately 51 to 74 percent of all individuals with COPD experience some level of depression.

With all of these issues to consider, you may wonder whether exercise is a good prescription for individuals with COPD. In fact, exercise can improve efficiency in ventilation, increase cardiovascular function, and increase muscle strength. All these benefits enhance breathing function and also help to decrease the anxiety related to dyspnea. Exercise is a required component in almost all pulmonary rehabilitation programs. Exercises that strengthen the arm and shoulder muscles not only help make breathing easier, but also provide functional independence. Exercise needs to be safe and customized to the individual's current level of COPD.

TABLE 1.5   SPECIAL NEEDS OF PARTICIPANTS WITH CHRONIC OBSTRUCTIVE PULMONARY DISEASE

Characteristic	Exercise and safety tips
Coughing attacks	Have the participant stop exercising. Encourage the participant to breathe slowly and try to relax.
Inability to breathe (dyspnea)	Have the participant stop exercising. Encourage the participant to keep an inhaler handy for use as needed. Be aware of any environmental toxins or pollutants in the room that may impair breathing function. Do not let participant drink any cold beverages, which may tighten the chest and make breathing more difficult. A warm drink may be more helpful.
Reduced stamina and endurance	Encourage rest periods to conserve energy and breath. Exercise routines should consist of short sessions of five to six exercise sets with one- to two-minute rests in between. The participant should start exercise slowly and eventually progress to exercising for 20 minutes if possible.
Shallow breathing	Avoid isometrics or weight above chest level. Encourage the participant to take it slowly and take breaks. Too many exercises with weights overhead increase blood pressure and increase the pressure in the chest, which makes breathing more difficult.
Oxygen use	Just knowing that oxygen is within reach gives some individuals the security to exercise. Be sure to provide adequate space for a portable oxygen tank during group exercise classes.
Anxiety and panic attacks	Be aware of signs and symptoms of emotional distress. If anxiety is causing any difficulty in breathing, remind the participant to anchor his or her arms and lean forward in a position of support. The participant can anchor the arms on the knees, a walker, a hand bar, or a similar support. This position helps the shoulders to support the upper body so that the chest is freer to expand, which allows more effective breathing. This position also gives the individual a sense of security and control. Encourage deep breathing and relaxation exercises (see chapters 4 and 7). Ask the participant if he or she would like you to place a fan with streamers attached to it nearby. Anxiety can be decreased by seeing air movement. Warm-up and cool-down exercises assist the respiratory system in acclimating to an increased activity level. This can help alleviate anxiety.

TABLE 1.6	SPECIAL NEEDS OF PARTICIPANTS WITH CORONARY ARTERY DISEASE
Characteristic	**Exercise and safety tips**
Lack of energy and endurance	Remind participant of the need to be consistent in exercising to increase energy and endurance.
Dizziness	The participant should warm up slowly and avoid sudden movements and changes in position.
Signs and symptoms of physical distress	Watch for these symptoms: chest discomfort, unusual shortness of breath, abnormal heart rhythm. If they occur, have the participant stop exercising immediately (refer to chapter 2, "Emergencies," page 29). Be sure that the room is not too cold or too hot.
Emotional stressors	Teach participant how to breathe deeply (see chapter 4). Encourage relaxation exercises (see chapter 7). Provide emotional support to participants who are experiencing anxiety about physical activity.
Difficulty breathing (dyspnea)	Remind participant to stop exercising and to breathe deeply and slowly. Be sure that the room is not too cold or too hot.

CORONARY ARTERY DISEASE

Coronary artery disease (CAD) occurs when the coronary arteries that supply blood to the heart muscle (myocardium) become progressively narrower. This narrowing of arteries is referred to as *atherosclerosis.* The narrowing is caused by atherosclerotic plaques, made up of fat and calcium, that form on the sides of the coronary artery wall, similar to those that cause ischemic stroke, and eventually cut off blood flow to the heart muscle.

The portion of the heart that is deprived of blood, and therefore oxygen, is said to be *ischemic* (deficient in blood). Ischemia causes pain, known as *angina pectoris.* This condition can progress and eventually cut off all blood flow to the heart muscle, causing a *myocardial infarction,* or heart attack. The damage can be mild, moderate, or severe, depending on the location and severity of the *infarct* (tissue death).

Coronary artery disease is greatly influenced by both genetics and lifestyle factors, such as diet, level of physical activity, stress, and smoking history. Anything that decreases atherosclerotic buildup decreases the risk of CAD. High blood pressure, high cholesterol, and diabetes can increase the risk of CAD.

Cardiac rehabilitation is offered after a myocardial infarction. Typically, cardiac rehabilitation takes place in three stages. Stage 1 begins in the hospital. The rehabilitation team works on basic skills of daily living. Stage 2 is done on an outpatient basis; the patient has returned home but goes to the hospital to participate in the rehabilitation program. Stage 3 is an individual program that the patient follows independently at home. This important stage significantly increases exercise endurance and tolerance (Ehsani 1987) and reduces the risk of subsequent heart attacks (O'Connor et al. 1989)

DEPRESSION

Depression is not a normal part of the aging process. It is classified as a mood disorder in the *Diagnostic and Statistical Manual of Mental Disorders* (DSM-IV; American Psychiatric Association 2000). This manual defines all currently recognized categories of mental disorders.

Mood is best described as *emotional content,* how someone feels, and it is influenced by various situations that a person encounters in everyday life. A mood disorder occurs when the cause of the mood is no longer as relevant as the impact of the mood on one's work, relationships, coping skills, and potential for happiness.

There are four diagnostic categories for depression: major depression (the most severe type), dysthymic disorder (milder depression with symptoms lasting over two years), adjustment disorder with depressed mood (a depressed mood resulting from a stressful event but that exceeds the normal reaction to such an event), and *bipolar disorder* (also known as manic-depressive illness, which is characterized by extreme mood swings).

Depression is the second most common mental disorder in long-term care settings, after dementia. It is estimated that 15 to 60 percent of older adults no longer living independently at home and those with significant health problems have clinically significant depressions (Cravern 1998).

TABLE 1.7 SPECIAL NEEDS OF PARTICIPANTS WITH DEPRESSION

Characteristic	Exercise and safety tips
Fatigue	Start slowly and establish easy-to-achieve and realistic goals.
Anger and frustration	Encourage participants to use exercise as a way to vent some of these feelings. A brisk walk or aerobic exercise of any type can help to alleviate some of these emotions. Group support is also beneficial in reducing some of these symptoms. Try to listen without giving advice or making judgments.
Negative outlook	Keep a positive attitude and encourage depressed individuals to participate. Remember to offer positive feedback and compliments. Try to keep your interaction with the participant lighthearted.
Difficulty with decision making	Be encouraging and involve participants in making decisions. Do not offer too many choices.
Insomnia	Ask participants how they slept the night before exercising. If they appear too fatigued, suggest a lighter workout than usual. Be observant for signs of overexertion. Encourage participants to spend time outside during the day, as sunshine helps improve the quality of sleep.
Decreased interest or pleasure in daily activities	Remind participant *in private* that this is a symptom of depression and that exercise can help. Also, encourage socializing with other members of the class.
Lack of sunlight stimulation	Many depressed individuals spend the majority of their day inside, away from sunlight. Sunlight not only improves the quality of sleep but also can decrease depression.
Lack of physical activity	Regular exercise (both aerobic and resistance training) is associated with increases in the brain chemicals endorphins and serotonin. Both of these can reduce the symptoms of depression.
Anxiety	Deep breathing (see chapter 4) and relaxation (see chapter 7) help decrease anxiety.

For many older people, the losses associated with age, illness, and change can bring about one of these types of depression. It is important to realize that over 80 percent of all depressions are treatable. In general, depression has clearly defined symptoms, but these vary among individuals. Depression must be diagnosed by a physician who has tested the individual. Many individuals experience the blues from a specific sad or traumatic event or even as a side effect from some medications. Others may not recognize that they are in a depression because they do not associate memory loss, lack of appetite, and especially sleep disturbances as symptoms. Depression is a complex illness. The good news is that exercise is an excellent intervention for all types of depression.

DIABETES

Diabetes is a chronic metabolic disorder that is characterized by a deficiency of insulin in the blood system. This deficiency results in hyperglycemia (an increase in blood sugar). Hyperglyce-mia can cause undue stress and damage to the kidneys, heart, nerves, eyes, and blood vessels. In addition, circulation is affected, which places an individual at risk of infection, especially in the legs and feet.

There are two categories of diabetes. Type 1 diabetes mellitus, or insulin-dependent, is identified as an absolute deficiency of insulin and can be diagnosed at any age. This type is insulin dependent and thought to be an autoimmune disorder. Of the 16 million people afflicted with diabetes, only 10 to 15 percent have type 1 diabetes.

Type 2 diabetes mellitus, or non-insulin-dependent (NIDDM), is the most prevalent and affects mostly older people, especially those who are obese. People with type 2 diabetes have a cellular resistance to insulin and may have reduced, normal, or elevated insulin levels. Of interest to the fitness leader is the fact that exercise and weight reduction, along with diet and medication, can improve blood glucose control in type 2 diabetes. Exercise has an insulin-like effect on the system in addition to reducing body fat. Over 75 percent of diabetics are at

TABLE 1.8 SPECIAL NEEDS OF PARTICIPANTS WITH DIABETES

Characteristic	Exercise and safety tips
Low tolerance to heat and cold	Avoid exercising in hot environments, as this increases the risk of heat injury for those with neuropathy (disease of the nerves). Avoid exercising in cold environments, which can impair circulation.
Poor circulation in legs and feet	Remind participants to wear comfortable and properly fitting shoes. Participants should be aware of positioning of feet and legs. Participants should avoid crossing the legs and feet.
Vision problems	Avoid exercises that can increase blood pressure (isometrics or too much exercise with arms overhead), which can harm the retinal blood vessels.
Potential for hypoglycemia (insulin reaction), the symptoms of which include faintness, sweating, dizziness, hunger, loss of motor coordination, rapid pulse, or confusion	See the section "Emergencies" in chapter 2 (page 29) and be sure to check the policies for medical emergencies specific to the setting that you teach in. Recommend that participant carry a medical ID.
Limited endurance	Remind participants to take breaks and not to overexert themselves.
Possible low blood sugar (type 1 diabetes)	Remind participant to check his or her blood sugar level before class. If it is low (under 70 milligrams per deciliter), the participant should eat a snack before any physical activity. The greater the physical activity, the more complex carbohydrates should be eaten. During exercise, blood glucose levels should be in the range of 100 to 250 milligrams per deciliter.
Taking beta blockers for heart problems	Be especially observant of participants who take these drugs, as they mask the symptoms of an insulin reaction.
Potential for dehydration	Remind participants to stop for water breaks.

higher risk of heart disease and stroke. Exercise can combat the buildup of LDL cholesterol (the artery-clogging agent), which increases with insulin resistance in the blood lipids.

The fitness leader should minimize the potential for hypoglycemic events among diabetic participants. Hypoglycemia (low blood sugar) occurs when there is too little glucose in the blood. The participant may have taken too much insulin, not eaten enough, or exercised too strenuously. The participant may feel hungry, weak, and dizzy and may tremble and perspire. This can become a very serious medical situation if not addressed immediately. A hypoglycemic person needs simple carbohydrates, such as orange juice or any sugary substance. Your observation makes all the difference in keeping individuals with diabetes exercising safely. See the section "Emergencies" in chapter 2 for a review of procedures if a medical emergency occurs during your exercise class.

HIP FRACTURE OR REPLACEMENT AND KNEE REPLACEMENT

Some participants in your exercise program may be receiving physical therapy for a hip fracture, a total or partial hip replacement, or knee replacement. The most important things to find out about those with hip and knee problems is how long it has been since their surgery, the precautions their physicians recommend, and how you can assist them in achieving therapy goals.

HYPERTENSION

Hypertension (high blood pressure) is considered a "silent killer" because, in its early stages, there are no symptoms. Any adult blood pressure over 140/90 is considered to be high. The 140 represents the *systolic blood pressure* (highest pressure in the arter-

TABLE 1.9 SPECIAL NEEDS OF PARTICIPANTS WITH HIP FRACTURE OR REPLACEMENT OR KNEE REPLACEMENT

Characteristic	Exercise and safety tips
Decreased functional mobility	Remind participant to move slowly and deliberately. Remind participants to be very aware of balance.
At risk of falls	Focus on safety in ambulation and transfers to and from a chair. Promote balance and strengthening exercises.
Pain	Participants should move only through a pain-free range of motion while exercising. Teach deep-breathing exercises along with relaxation techniques for pain management and reduction (see chapters 4 and 7).
For total and partial hip replacements	To prevent hip dislocation, the participant should follow these recommendations unless his or her physician or physical therapist recommends otherwise: Do not bend at hip more than 90 degrees. Avoid sitting in low-seated chairs. Keep knees lower than the hips. Do not cross the legs. Avoid internal rotation (pointing the toes inward).
For total knee replacement	Pain can be a problem with knee replacements. Follow the pain tips given earlier. There are no limitations on upper-body exercising. The participant may be able to bear full weight with no limitations on exercise.

TABLE 1.10 SPECIAL NEEDS OF PARTICIPANTS WITH HYPERTENSION

Characteristic	Exercise and safety tips
Shortness of breath	Offer frequent rest periods; participants should not overexert themselves.
Limited endurance	Aerobic exercises are encouraged, as they reduce systolic blood pressure and also help to increase endurance. However, high-intensity exercise should be discouraged.
Increased blood pressure with exercise	Avoid continuous over-the-head work with or without weights, as this increases blood pressure.
General recommendations	People with blood pressure over 180/110 should begin drug treatment before beginning endurance training (ACSM 1997). Stress reduction and relaxation exercises (see chapter 7) decrease blood pressure and should be encouraged. Remind participants to breath while exercising so that blood pressure does not get elevated. Isometric exercises should be avoided, as they can elevate blood pressure.

ies at any time) and 90, the *diastolic blood pressure* (lowest pressure in the arteries at any time). When the blood pressure is higher than average, the heart needs to work harder. This stresses the heart and puts a greater demand on the arteries. Possible consequences include enlargement of the heart and arteriosclerosis (hardening of the arteries). Hypertension also increases the risk of stroke.

Some of the causes of hypertension are related to lifestyle and diet. In addition, some medications, such as birth control pills, steroids, decongestants, and anti-inflammatories, increase the risk of high blood pressure (Kaiser Permanente 1994).

The origin of some cases of hypertension is unknown. In such cases, physicians often request that patients cut back on sodium and fats in their diets and add moderate exercise to their weekly schedules. These lifestyle modifications help physicians to further evaluate the origin of the hypertension and then decide on the necessary treatment.

One known risk factor is inactivity. Exercise is a positive intervention for hypertension. A moderate-intensity program (below 70 percent of maximum heart rate) is recommended to decrease both systolic and diastolic blood pressure (Brooks, Fahey, and White 1996).

Multiple Sclerosis

Multiple sclerosis (MS) is a progressive and degenerative neurologic disorder. It affects the central nervous system. An insulating fatty sheath, called myelin, protects the nerve fibers in a healthy person. With MS, this protecting layer is damaged, which consequently impairs the function of the affected nerves in the brain and spinal cord.

Like most diseases, MS differs in different people. It can be mild or severe; there can be remissions for years or no remissions. This disease afflicts young to middle-aged adults. More women than men are affected. The origin of the disorder is unknown.

An individual with MS may need a wheelchair for mobility. As the disease progresses, people with MS may need assistance with all activities of daily living. It is not uncommon for a young person with MS to live in a long-term care facility because of the complexity of his or her needs. Along with their physical limitations, many individuals with MS have emotional difficulties related to their loss of independence and function.

TABLE 1.11	SPECIAL NEEDS OF PARTICIPANTS WITH MULTIPLE SCLEROSIS
Characteristic	**Exercise and safety tips**
Inability to tolerate heat	Locate the participant close to ventilation. Avoid exercising in hot environments.
Limited energy reserve	Remind participants to take breaks. Teach energy-conservation techniques. Participants with limited energy need to prioritize physical activities.
Decreased coordination (increased risk of falls)	Keep the environment safe and clear of obstacles. Provide space between seats. Do not hurry from one movement to another. Allow extra time to move from one exercise position to another. Keep exercise movements simple.
Possible vision deficits	Locate the participant close to the leader. Use contrasting colors for instructional materials, as the participant may have problems with color discrimination. Keep the environment free from clutter.
Loss of feeling in limbs, numbness, tingling (paresthesia)	Be aware of participant's body positioning in chair, as the participant may not detect sitting incorrectly. Observe placement of feet and hands to avoid injury.
Spasticity (including foot drag, stiffness, or lack of control of one or both legs), muscle weakness, potentially limited range of motion	Begin exercises slowly as participant may be deconditioned and weakened in addition to experiencing spastic weakness. All movements should be slow. Avoid too much work by any one muscle group. Eliminate neck exercises if participant has any weakness or loss of control of neck muscles.
Possible impairment of respiratory function	Be aware of any breathing difficulties. If they are observed, have participant stop exercising.
Decreased range of motion	Never force any stretch or movement. Remind participant always to move within a pain-free range of motion.
Loss of muscular coordination in trunk or limbs (ataxia)	Encourage participants to keep arms close to their sides, which can alleviate some tremors.

OSTEOPOROSIS

Osteoporosis is a disease that is characterized by low bone density. This density loss leads to brittle and porous bones. Osteoporosis is a major health threat to over 28 million Americans, 80 percent of whom are women. Osteoporosis is considered a silent epidemic because the disease is often not detected in the early stages (although a bone-density test can offer early detection) until there are visible signs, such as loss of height, a forward-curved upper back, or broken bones in the hip, wrist, or spine. The more visible the signs, the more advanced the disease. Many individuals have some degree of lowered bone mass *(osteopenia),* which is considered the precursor to osteoporosis. As the body ages, there are some natural declines in bone mass. In addition,

loss of bone mass can be due to a lack of physical activity or a lack of calcium in the diet.

Osteoporosis is a disease affecting primarily postmenopausal women. Osteoporosis among menopausal women is due to a decrease in estrogen levels. As estrogen levels decrease, bone thinning and bone loss occur. Most of the bone loss occurs in the early stages of menopause. Postmenopausal women have less bone loss, but they may still be losing more bone than their systems replace. Other individuals experience bone loss caused by the use of steroid medications, vitamin and mineral deficiencies, heavy drinking, smoking, a thin and small-framed body, and not enough weight-bearing exercise.

Regardless of the cause of bone loss, postmenopausal women are at higher risk of bone fractures

TABLE 1.12 SPECIAL NEEDS OF PARTICIPANTS WITH OSTEOPOROSIS

Characteristic	Exercise and safety tips
Kyphosis, need for sensory input, increased risk of falling	Avoid exercises that increase *spinal flexion* (bending forward at the waist). This position can increase risk of vertebral fractures. Avoid overload of the back. Be aware of safety hazards in the environment, as participants may not have a clear view of surroundings due to their posture. Provide exercises that bring the shoulders back, expand the chest, and enhance the participant's ability to stand straighter, stronger, and with better balance. This can be very encouraging for an individual with kyphosis.
Bone fractures	Fractures can occur spontaneously with decalcified (brittle) bones (osteoporotic fractures). Avoid exercises that involve leaning forward over the knees, particularly in combination with stooping over. Fast, jerky movements should be avoided at all times. Remind participants to always sit slowly and stay in control of their movements.
Anxiety	Because of the risk of fractures, many individuals are anxious about becoming physically active. They need emotional support and a safe environment in which to exercise.
Chronic back pain	Seated resistance exercises are encouraged, as they help build muscle strength and prevent falls while exercising. If approved, standing resistance and weight-bearing exercises can help increase both bone density and back strength.
Risk of falling	Avoid any exercises that impair balance. Encourage a good seated posture. Remind participants always to wear shoes that have a nonskid bottom. Exercises should focus on building up the larger muscle groups so as to cushion a fall if it occurs.
Stiffness	Always have participants start exercising slowly to warm up the joints and muscles.
Fatigue	A stooped position can impair the participant's pulmonary function and thus limit endurance. Watch for signs of fatigue, and encourage participants to rest between exercises as needed. Self-monitoring is important. Participants need to stop when they feel too fatigued.

TABLE 1.13	SPECIAL NEEDS OF PARTICIPANTS WITH PARKINSON'S DISEASE
Characteristic	**Exercise and safety tips**
Resting tremors	Holding light weights and relaxation techniques (see chapter 7) help decrease tremors.
Rigidity	Reciprocal (moving backward and forward) and rotational (turning on an axis) physical exercises help decrease rigidity.
Stooped posture	Remind participants often to be aware of their posture. Encourage exercises such as backward shoulder rotation.
Slow movements (bradykinesia)	Take extra time to complete each movement. Have the participant warm up muscles slowly and change positions slowly. Break exercises into steps.
Postural instability	Frequently remind participants to be aware of their posture. Encourage the participant to walk with larger steps and try to lift the foot off the floor with each step. A good posture exercise is standing with one's back against a wall, with the back of the head (if possible, while keeping the chin level), shoulders, buttocks, calves, and heels touching the wall, while envisioning good posture.
Acceleration or abbreviation of walking movements (festination)	When festination occurs, have the participant stop, breathe, and reposture before beginning to walk again. Remind the participant to allow a good space between the feet for balance before walking.
Uncontrolled movements (dyskinesia) and shaking movement of limbs (ataxia)	Physical activity can help reduce dyskinesia and ataxia. While seated, have participant follow your movements: Stretch arms out in front of chest, clench fists, and release. Slowly bring arms to sides, and shake them out. Breathe deeply.
Freezing of movements	If freezing occurs during ambulation, have participant stop moving, ensure good distance between feet, slowly sway from side to side, and then proceed with walking. Sometimes the side-to-side movements of dancing can help to break the freeze. This dancing should be tried only on a one-on-one basis. Walking is a recommended physical activity. Marching in place is a good variation. Chair exercises and slow stretching exercises are also advised.
Motor problems, motor memory problems	Repeat directions and follow up with visual demonstrations. Participants should exercise slowly without any jerky movements.
Difficulty with oral or facial control	Speech can become faint and facial expressions may lessen. To combat both of these, include breathing exercises (e.g., pronouncing "AEIOU," smiling, singing, and whistling).
Dementia	Use visual cues to teach exercises. Break exercises into easy steps. Keep it simple.
Depression	Focus on the abilities and functions that the participant still has. Exercise, social connectedness, and having fun help to decrease symptoms of depression.

due to osteoporosis. When the bones are weakened, the potential for injury during exercise increases. The majority of fractures take place in the vertebrae, hips, and wrists.

A participant may have severe spinal deformity that impedes his or her ability to stand up straight (kyphosis). This condition can be the result of osteoporosis. Because kyphosis impairs bal-ance and alters the center of gravity, the risk of falling increases. Kyphosis can also alter respiratory function because of the confinement of the chest.

Many participants in your class may have some level of osteoporosis or osteopenia. It is estimated that 90 percent of residents of long-term care facilities have osteoporosis. This high percentage causes

TABLE 1.14	SPECIAL NEEDS OF PARTICIPANTS WITH SENSORY LOSSES
Characteristic	**Exercise and safety tips**
Vision loss	Use large print for written materials. Remember to always use dark-colored print on a white background for ideal contrast. Remember that your verbal description and verbal pacing dictate how participants learn the exercises. Participants with vision loss have greater sensitivity to light and may take longer to adjust to changes in light levels. Avoid clutter in the environment. When sitting down, participants should feel the chair with their hands for proper positioning.
Glaucoma	Avoid any position that increases blood flow to or fluid in the eyes.
Hearing loss (often a hidden, or undetected, disability)	Remember to speak at a normal volume. Do not shout. Keep the pitch of your voice normal, and make direct eye contact with the listener. Music playing in the background can be both an annoyance and a distraction from exercising safely. Be visually demonstrative so that participants can use your body language as a cue. Use gestures. Rephrase your directions if they are not clearly understood. Remind participants who wear hearing aides to bring the arms close to the ears but not touch them when such movements are required in an exercise.
Communication losses, including expressive aphasia (inability to express oneself), receptive aphasia (inability to receive information clearly), or global aphasia (both)	Make directions simple, and visually demonstrate them. Give participants positive feedback on their performance.
Loss of sensation	Participants may not feel heat, cold, or pain in their hands or feet, and so should keep them in a safe position.

1.5 million fractures yearly (California Department of Health Services, Institute for Health and Aging; California Osteoporosis Prevention and Education Program 1998). Exercise is a very important intervention in this disorder. Although osteoporosis is not reversible, exercise can at least slow down the age- and inactivity-related decline in bone mass (ACSM 1995).

PARKINSON'S DISEASE

Parkinson's disease is a degenerative and progressive neurologic disorder. The disease affects both movement and posture. Neurotransmitters within the brain help relay signals from the peripheral nervous system to the brain. The neurotransmitter dopamine is significantly reduced or destroyed in this disease process. The symptoms related to this reduction are resting tremors, slow movements

(bradykinesia), postural instability, uncontrolled movements *(dyskinesia)*, involuntary cessation of a movement *(freezing)*, gait disorders, and shuffling. There are also changes in the volume of the voice. In some cases dementia is related to this disorder.

SENSORY LOSSES

Many older adults are living with one or more sensory losses, such as loss of vision, hearing, or sensation. Singularly or in any combination, these losses additionally challenge an individual who is attempting to master the environment and stay functionally independent.

It is important for you to be aware of any sensory limitations a participant has to ensure that the participant can exercise safely to his or her full potential. Some strategies for teaching participants with sensory losses are reviewed in chapter 3.

TRAUMATIC HEAD INJURY

Traumatic head injury occurs when the head collides with another surface. This collision causes the brain to impact on the inside of the skull. In addition to the direct brain injury, a head trauma may incur other injuries, such as *edema* (an excessive amount of tissue fluid) and *ischemia* (a local and temporary deficiency of blood supply due to obstruction of the circulation to a body part).

The victim of a head injury can be any age, although those between the ages of 15 to 24 and 75 and over are more prone to such injuries. The major-ity are young accident victims. Directly after a head trauma, a medical team should assess the injury to determine whether it is mild, moderate, or severe. If cognitive impairments are mild to moderate, the patient may need only acute medical assistance. If the impairment is moderate to severe, the individual may have a chronic disorder and need specialized long-term care.

Some of the symptoms of a traumatic head injury are agitation, confusion, short attention span, short- and long-term memory loss, and combativeness. Because of these problems, it is important to keep this individual in a calm environment with few

TABLE 1.15 SPECIAL NEEDS OF PARTICIPANTS WITH TRAUMATIC HEAD INJURY	
Characteristic	**Exercise and safety tips**
Poor judgment	Keep the environment structured and directions simple to follow.
Disinhibition	Maintain a low-stimulus environment. Set limits for appropriate and inappropriate behavior in a social setting.
	It may be necessary to gently remove participant from the group and work with him or her one-on-one if possible.
Possible hemiparesis	Encourage participant to work with the affected side by having the strong arm help move the affected arm or leg in exercises.
	Be aware of participants' positioning in the chair during seated exercises, as they may not be able to feel whether they are sitting safely.
	Remind the participant to keep the affected arm on the lap for protection and avoid letting it hang over the side of the chair.
Poor balance and coordination	Encourage participants to focus on their posture while sitting in a chair. They should sit all the way back in the chair. If they fall to one side or their affected arm hangs over the side of the chair, verbally remind them to reposition. Have them use the strong hand to pick up the affected arm and place it in their lap.
	Use exercises that involve both sides of the body. They enhance balance and coordination. Exercise movements that take the participant off the midline or center of balance help build balance control. Some exercise ideas are ball toss or kicking. Trying to catch a ball on their affected side enhances both balance and body awareness.
Difficulty planning and carrying out movements	Keep movements simple. All movements and follow-through deserve positive feedback.
	Hand-over-hand assistance may be necessary. Ask permission to help, and approach participant slowly while making eye contact.
Perceptual problems	Help participants more easily differentiate between the foreground and background of signs and written materials by using strong color contrast, such as black and white.
Speech and language problems	Speak clearly and give very simple directions.
	Look directly at the participant. Give him or her extra time to respond.
Overstimulation	Balance active and passive behaviors in the exercise class. The participant needs frequent breaks to stay relaxed.
Frustration with potential for aggression and catastrophic reactions	Because frustration is a common emotional response due to head injury, do not overchallenge participants. They need to feel successful in performing very simple steps.

distractions. In an exercise class, keep space between them and equipment or other participants so that they do not harm themselves or others.

SUMMARY

The population of older adults is increasing at a faster rate than any other age group. Most older adults in exercise classes in certain settings have special needs or some level of frailty. Depending on their functional needs, adults who are frail or who have special needs may live independently or in a variety of assisted-living or special care facilities. Regardless of older adults' level of need, physical activity is their best way to preserve physical function and independence. The MacArthur Foundation 10-year study of aging verified that genes are only one of many factors that play a role in living well as we age (Rowe and Kahn 1998).

Inactivity is one of our greatest obstacles. Inactivity plays a major role in cardiovascular problems, high blood pressure, pulmonary disorders, depression, diabetes, and osteoporosis. It also can be a contributing factor to other health problems. Even moderate exercise can make a big difference. The U.S. Surgeon General's report called *Physical Activity and Health* (1996) considers physical activity so important that it is identified as a national *call to action*.

Today's fitness leaders are answering this call. They are knowledgeable about the special needs of their audience, and their exercise classes are designed on a firm base of professional and safety standards. By following the guidelines and recommendations in this book, you can not only teach your audience about lifestyle and health issues, but also learn important lessons for yourself as you age. Focus on function, fitness, and fun.

CHAPTER 2

THE EXERCISE PROGRAM: MAKE IT MOTIVATING, SAFE, AND EFFECTIVE

Physical exercise is important for all individuals regardless of their limitations or existing health conditions. This message was one of the key points in a report by the U.S. Surgeon General (1996). From this report and the growing interest in physical activity in older persons, the U.S. Department of Health and Human Services (2000) designed the *Healthy People 2010* objectives and the National Institute on Aging created the *National Blueprint: Increasing Physical Activity Among Adults Age 50 and Older* (AARP et al. 2001). Specifically, these reports state the need for all communities, agencies, and businesses to promote physical activity among their members and for all individuals to become more physically active both to increase quality of life and to decrease the health care needs of our aging population.

Whether you are a seasoned fitness instructor or new to the field, this chapter walks you through a few of the most important areas in developing a safe and effective exercise program.

The exercise program provided in part II is designed to be customized with the individual participant in mind. When working with the frail elderly and adults with special needs, you must observe and assess their abilities and limitations and consistently evaluate their need for exercise modifications. Additionally, you need to hone your motivational skills so that participants are encouraged to keep coming back to your classes.

This chapter looks at how to motivate participants, adhere to safety guidelines and industry standards, and incorporate our experience into your exercise program.

MAKE IT MOTIVATING

Do you ever wonder what draws people to an exercise class, and what makes it a success? Participants attend for various reasons. Some are encouraged by family, therapists, or facility staff to attend exercise programs. Others come because they seek social interaction. And some attend because they have always been physically active and are continuing to pursue their interest. Most people come looking for experiences other than strictly exercise.

IMPORTANCE OF MOTIVATION

Motivation is the force that initially brings participants to your class and brings them back. Personal motivation is a very powerful tool. Fitness leaders need to be aware of each participant's motivation and goals. This awareness gives fitness leaders better insight into who the participant is, what he or she needs from them, and how to personalize the exercise program.

Participants may be motivated to achieve intrinsic or extrinsic goals. Intrinsic goals come from within the individual. For example, I may want to join an exercise class because I want to lose weight or try something new. These are self-directed motivators—intrinsic goals. Extrinsic goals are external motivators. For example, I may pursue training to achieve a certificate or award.

Extrinsic motivators vary over the stages of our lives. However, the intrinsic motivators give us the staying power to continue. Both the intrinsic and the extrinsic motivators are important. At times, people may need more external motivators to keep them going until they feel the internal benefits from the experience.

As the leader of the fitness class, you should find ways to help motivate each participant intrinsically or extrinsically. You first need to persuade participants to come and to participate in the exercise class. Continuity and frequency of exercise can help your participants see and feel the personal benefits of physical activity. Seeing and feeling these benefits can increase participants' motivation if their individual goals are being met. When participants experience success and notice how their exercising has affected their day-to-day life, be sure to have them share their story with the class. It is always uplifting and motivating to hear about others' successes.

Creating realistic goals for each participant is crucial for motivation. The next section presents some points to remember in creating goals with and for your participants.

GOAL SETTING

You can instill confidence in your participants by assisting them in identifying and achieving their goals. Many older adults have not established goals for fitness. You can help them determine their goals. Individuals who set specific health- and exercise-related goals better adhere to their programs. Individuals who also identify realistic fitness goals have more success in achieving them. We recommend that you have participants identify and write down their first fitness goal. This goal is first created with the leader and individual participant. It is written on the Medical History and Risk Factor Questionnaire (appendix E). A copy of this is kept by the fitness leader and also the participant upon request. In addition, it is added to the Fitness Leader's Log form (next page). The Fitness Goal Map (appendix H), a light-hearted cartoon, can be customized with the participant's short- and long-term goals filled in on the road signs (as shown in the figure below). This appendix is meant to be fun and easy to use. This should be kept by the participant and a copy could be kept by the leader also. For some of your participants, the questionnaire form will be sufficient. For others, the Fitness Goal Map will be additional.

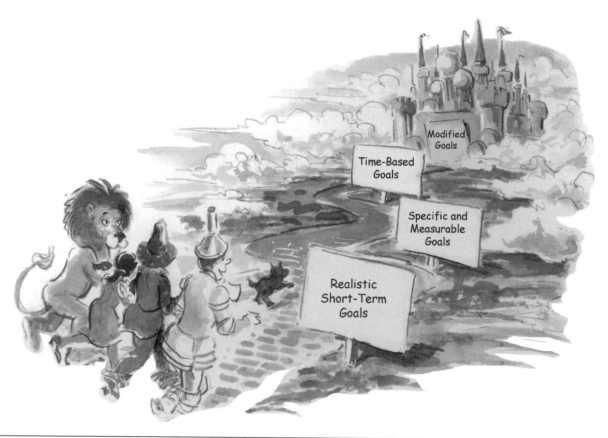

Fitness goal map.

Adapted, by permission, from S.N. Blair, et al., 2001, *Active living everyday* (Champaign, IL: Human Kinetics), 55.

FITNESS LEADER'S LOG

Name:

_____

Diagnosis:

_____

Medications:

_____

Physician's or physical therapist's special recommendations:

_____

Exercise clearance forms completed: ❏ Informed consent ❏ Questionnaire ❏ Medical clearance form ❏ PAR-Q

Contact person and phone number:

Comments	Date	Fitness and modified goal(s)

These are qualities of good fitness goals:

- Realistic (i.e., achievable) for the individual
- Specific and measurable (The more concrete the goal is, the easier it is to measure success.)
- Time-based, to provide some schedule in which to work (Goals may be short or long term.)
- Easily modified if and when circumstances change

Let's look more closely at these four areas of fitness goal setting.

• Setting realistic goals. Some participants want to achieve goals that are not realistic for them at the time. The fitness leader should encourage them to be realistic and truthful in setting goals and expectations. Help them set goals that can be achieved and then built upon. For example, one of your participants, Mr. Judd, tells you that he wants to start walking again without a walker. Remember that the goal needs to be realistic, and encourage him to discuss the goal of walking without a walker with his physician or physical therapist. The physician or therapist may then send a note to you requesting a focus on specific exercises that reinforce their treatment or therapy goals. From this information and your assessment and observations, you can better define and clarify realistic fitness goals. The medical clearance form and cover letter to the physician should help you gather and document helpful information for goal setting. Example of a realistic goal: Mr. Judd will participate in a seated exercise program two to three times a week to increase his activity level and learn the chair stand.

• Setting specific and measurable goals. Goals help the participant see his or her progress step by step. Break the larger goal into obtainable steps. Mr. Judd may not currently be able to walk without a walker, but it may be a long-term goal if approved by his physician. That is why we start with obtaining the physician's approval. If this is not a realistic goal, we help the participant identify more realistic goals to work toward. It is also important for the fitness leader to realize that each different setting will have varying protocols for how they obtain the physician's approval, establish goals, and work with the individual participant. By breaking the goal of walking unaided into the short-term goals of strengthening specific muscles, for example, a participant can look for small changes and experience success. Remember that the more specific the goal, the easier it is to measure success and progress. Example of a specific and measurable goal: Mr. Judd

will participate in a resistance-training program three times a week with a special focus on building strength in his quadriceps, hamstrings, and triceps to successfully complete a chair stand.

• Setting time-based goals. Change takes time. Participants should begin exercising slowly. Never rush fitness goals. Determine how much time is needed to see the benefits of the exercises. Keep breaking goals down into obtainable steps, and keep participants working on short-term goals first. This gives them small successes along the way to obtaining long-term fitness goals. It is not important to establish a specific date, but rather to project how long you anticipate that they will be working on a specific goal. With this timeline, the participant and you can evaluate progress and, if necessary, reassess the goal. Use your attendance records to visually reinforce how long a participant has been involved in exercising. Example of a time-based goal: Mr. Judd will be able to successfully complete a chair stand with chair-arm assistance in three months.

• Modifying the goals. The frail elderly and adults with special needs can experience fatigue, lack of sleep, changes in vision and hearing, new medical conditions, emotional or memory difficulties, and other changes that negatively affect their exercise participation and abilities. These changes can be discouraging to the participant and can alter fitness goals. By redefining goals together, you can help the participant succeed at his or her level of ability. One fitness goal may be simply to maintain the current frequency, intensity, and duration of exercises. Goal setting is a cyclic process. When change occurs, you reevaluate the goal, make sure it is realistic for the participant's new level or need, make it specific and measurable, and then set a new schedule. The following is an example of a modified goal: Because of a new diagnosis of Parkinson's disease and associated tremors, Mr. Judd will *maintain* his current goal of an arm-assisted chair stand for the next three to six months rather than *progressing* to an independent chair stand. Maintaining current functional levels versus progressing them is a good and realistic goal for many frail elderly participants. It is important to discuss these issues with them individually. You will find that most participants are realistic and listen closely to your recommendations.

You can keep track of these changes on the Fitness Leader's Log form. Significant changes can also be noted on the medical history questionnaire. Once fitness goals are established, remind participants of all the benefits of their hard work in exercising. These reminders are both motivational and educational to the participant.

BENEFITS OF EXERCISE

Some participants in your class may be very physically active, and others may continue to live very sedentary lives. In addition, many of your participants may be dealing with multiple medical disorders along with physical frailties. The benefits of exercise may not be easy for them to see in the beginning. Part of your role as fitness leader is to educate your participants about the benefits of exercise. You need to help them see how these are relevant to their own lives and health. One of the best ways to make exercise relevant is to correlate an exercise with an everyday function. Table 6.5 in chapter 6 gives examples of the functional roles of resistance exercises.

One example of a functional role (or benefit) of a resistance exercise is walking up the stairs. When the correlation is clear, the participant can see why strengthening specific lower-extremity muscles such as the quadriceps will benefit them. Another example is looking behind you, as if to see who is calling you from behind. From a seated position, this movement takes flexibility to twist and rotate the head toward the shoulder. Flexibility and stretching exercises enhance the participant's ability to look over the shoulder. Lifting objects and reaching for objects are other examples that you can use. When participants are able to recognize these exercise benefits for themselves, the benefits become intrinsic motivators. This makes the exercise program relevant for the individual participant.

Promoting independence and maintaining or improving function are two of the greatest benefits and goals of an exercise program for frail elders and adults with special needs. By seeing an improvement in physical endurance and strength, a participant can begin to see himself or herself as a more active and vital person. This perception can transform a previously sedentary individual into an active and more independent person.

Lists of physiological and psychological benefits from the World Health Organization (1997) appear in appendixes A and B. You can make copies of these charts and hand them out to your participants. You can refer to them often and also post enlarged copies in the exercise room for reference. These educational handouts can be very motivating.

In addition to being motivating and effective, your exercise class needs to be safe. The following section presents some ways to make all aspects of your class safe.

MAKE IT SAFE

At any age, physical exercise carries risks. As an instructor working with frail elders and adults with special needs, you need to know your participants' limitations, their established goals, and any exercises that are contraindicated for them. Concern for safety not only helps you be a better teacher, but it also instills confidence in your participants. Frail elderly people have fears of failing, falling, and looking foolish. Being assured of safety builds confidence, security, and competence and overcomes these initial anxieties related to physical activity.

Safety starts with knowing your participants. The first step is obtaining medical clearance from their physicians.

MEDICAL CLEARANCE

The responsibility of the fitness leader is to know and understand each participant's abilities and limitations. The first source of information about these issues is the physician. Every participant should have a physician who oversees his or her health. The initial step in making exercise safe is to request information regarding health issues and limitations from the physician.

The Statement of Medical Clearance for Exercise in appendix C is a sample form for the physician to complete to give the participant clearance to take part in the exercise program. Review this form and feel free to adapt it to suit your setting and program. This form can be faxed or mailed to the physician's office. If the physician feels an individual has too many medical issues to address in a classroom setting, the physician may not give his or her approval. The form also includes a comments section, where the physician can write in any limitations or cautionary notes for the fitness leader. Appendix D is a sample cover letter that you can fax or mail to the physician with the medical clearance form. Note any details about contraindicated exercises or limitations on the completed form, then file it.

ASSESSMENT

As mentioned in the earlier section on motivation, your participants come to exercise class for personal reasons. Regardless of their motivations for attending, you need to clearly understand their current limitations, medical conditions, and ability levels. Without this information, you cannot ensure that their fitness goals are safe and appropriate. There are many types of forms to assess an individual's fitness level and needs. We suggest using some or all of the following questionnaires.

• A Medical History and Risk Factor Questionnaire (appendix E) allows the fitness leader to gather information about the current physical status of an individual participant. This questionnaire is a tool to use in the evaluation for establishing fitness goals. The Medical History and Risk Factor Questionnaire records both past and current health issues. It also identifies any current functional limitations and fitness goals. If you do not currently have a form to use, feel free to adapt this form to your program needs.

• We also recommend that you have each participant complete the Exercise Program Informed Consent form found in appendix F. By signing this form, participants state that they consent to participate and understand the risks of the program. This form is completed along with requesting the physician's approval.

• The PAR-Q and You fitness questionnaire (appendix G) is another widely used form designed to assess an individual's readiness to begin exercising. If a respondent answers yes to one or more of the questions, be sure to have that person check with the doctor before starting the exercise program. We recommend always obtaining the physician's approval as a safety guideline.

If you are not using a standard form, be sure that you gather the information shown in the checklist below during the assessment.

The assessment process always begins with your initial interview and conversation with a partici-

pant. In this interview, you will begin to gather the information needed to assess this participant's strengths, limitations, and goals for joining.

The Medical History and Risk Factor Questionnaire form records an informational baseline: where the participant started from along with previous medical history and initial fitness goals. All other observations and records are compared with this initial baseline. If you create a progress or attendance board, the results of testing are recorded by date. Such a board, which is an extrinsic motivator, visually conveys a participant's progress.

It is important to understand that the assessment process varies from setting to setting according to participants' functional abilities and ability to live independently. Some fitness leaders teach and assess participants in more than one setting. You may gather some or all of this information listed earlier depending on the protocols and procedures of the setting of your program.

ASSESSMENT IN RETIREMENT COMMUNITIES AND SENIOR CENTERS

In a life-care or other retirement community or community senior center, you may lead exercises for physically active and independent elderly participants. For instance, participants may live in their own houses or apartments and may receive assistance with some areas of daily living. Their level of assistance is important for you to know. For example, a participant may live at home but receive physical therapy for injuries from a recent fall or a

Assessment Checklist

❑ Initial interview

❑ Previous lifestyle and exercise information

❑ Review of medical and social history

❑ Identification of existing conditions

❑ Identification of previous injuries and conditions

❑ Physician's approval and recommendations or precautions

❑ Therapeutic recommendations and precautions

❑ Results and information from any previous fitness testing

From *Exercise for Frail Elders* by E. Best-Martini and K. A. Botenhagen-DiGenova, 2003, Champaign, IL: Human Kinetics.

recent fracture. The participant may have someone helping with food preparation and temporarily helping him or her to transfer from a chair to bed, and so on. Participants of an exercise class at a senior center also may have special needs that are not visible to you. During the initial assessment, be sure to ask about areas of personal care with which they need assistance. Their answers will help you understand their current level of physical functioning.

ASSESSMENT IN ASSISTED-LIVING OR RESIDENTIAL CARE FACILITIES, ADULT DAY HEALTH CENTERS, OR SKILLED NURSING SETTINGS

Specific federal and state regulations require that exercise programs be offered in assisted-living or residential care settings (the residents of which need some level of assistance with activities of daily living), adult day health centers (a day program that provides nursing supervision, therapists, and social workers), and skilled nursing settings (convalescent care). Residents live in or regularly visit these settings for some medical reason. They may have limitations in activities of daily living or memory loss that prevents them from living alone. Adult day health programs have physical, occupational, speech, and recreation therapists on staff along with social workers and activity directors to provide a medical model—a medical team approach. These settings provide you with much support for exercise assessment.

Those in skilled nursing settings need 24-hour nursing supervision. Participants are often in frail physical condition and depend on staff for one or more of their activities of daily living. The staff in these settings may already have a form for assessing *functional fitness* (a person's ability to perform daily activities) and for requesting the physician's approval. Because the approach to care in skilled nursing facilities is interdisciplinary, they also provide you with support in the assessment process.

SAFETY GUIDELINES

Let's look at safety issues in the exercise class. Both the leader and the participants have many safety issues to consider. The "Safety Guidelines Checklist" on page 30 can serve as a quick reminder and adds to your safety awareness. It is broken into two parts, one for the leader and the other for the participants. These lists emphasize that the responsibility for exercise safety lies with both the leader and the participant. Additionally, chapters 4 through 7 in part II have a "Safety Precautions" section. Each section offers safety tips specific to each component of an exercise program.

EMERGENCIES

One of the fitness leader's most important safety responsibilities is dealing with medical and other emergencies. As the fitness instructor, you need to have an emergency plan in case something unexpected happens. Request a copy of the emergency policy and procedures from the staff at the facility where you teach. The policy and procedures both for medical emergencies and for natural disasters are important for you to know. The policy should outline the command structure in an emergency. You should know exactly who to call on-site if an emergency occurs in your class. If no such policy is in place, design a simple plan of action to follow in case of any emergency in the classroom. Depending on the setting, many fitness leaders carry their own first-aid kit with them to class.

We recommend that you have both a completed Medical History and Risk Factor Questionnaire (appendix E) and a signed physician's approval form (appendix C) for each of your participants. Keep a log on each participant that includes the information gathered from both of these forms. Know not only their diagnoses and previous medical histories but also what medications they are taking. Many medications have side effects that can alter mood, balance, and coordination. Knowing this information can make all the difference in an emergency. On the log, be sure to note a contact person and phone number for each participant. Many of the settings for exercise classes, including retirement communities, day centers, and hospitals, have these records available. If not, use the form Fitness Leader's Log to keep all this information together.

Along with information about individual participants, familiarize yourself with the environment in which you teach. Look around for the items in the emergency checklist on page 31.

In an emergency you should know what to do first. In a crisis situation, try to determine the severity of the incident. Does someone need to call 911? Remember that someone else on-site may be responsible for calling 911. Your role may be to immediately bring in the on-site nursing or administrative staff to determine the response needed. This staff member may be able to handle the crisis right then or may make the decision to call 911.

Safety Guidelines Checklist

Safety Guidelines for the Leader

❑ Be sure that each participant has medical clearance from his or her physician.

❑ Be sure that all participants breathe continuously during the exercises. Holding one's breath can increase blood pressure.

❑ Watch for signs of overfatigue or other indications that the activity level is too demanding.

❑ Avoid too many exercises that involve overhead movements. Continuously raising or holding the arms overhead (especially while holding weight) can raise blood pressure.

❑ Be vigilant while teaching. Always monitor how participants respond to the exercise.

❑ Exercise should never cause pain. Have a participant stop exercising if he or she experiences any pain.

❑ Avoid combining any resistance exercises with exercises that involve turning or bending the spine.

❑ Avoid teaching full neck rotations. Each head and neck movement should be completed separately and slowly.

❑ Be aware of the environment and any potential safety hazards (including a room that is too hot or too cold).

❑ Ask your participants how they felt after the last workout the next time you see them so that you can give them appropriate guidance for the next class.

Safety Guidelines for the Participant

❑ Be aware of your posture in a chair or a wheelchair.

❑ Do not try to compete with other participants. Everyone needs to exercise at his or her own pace and within his or her own ability.

❑ Avoid jerking or thrusting movements while exercising.

❑ During standing exercises, be sure to hold on to a steady chair, a hand rail, or the wall for safety.

❑ During seated exercises, do not raise both feet off the ground at the same time. This can add undue stress to your back.

❑ When you are leaning or bending forward during a seated exercise, be sure to support yourself by placing your hands on your knees.

❑ Prevent dehydration; take water breaks during the exercise class.

❑ Don't overdo it. Mild muscle soreness lasting up to a few days and slight fatigue are normal. What are not normal are exhaustion, sore joints, and unpleasant muscle soreness.

 From *Exercise for Frail Elders* by E. Best-Martini and K. A. Botenhagen-DiGenova, 2003, Champaign, IL: Human Kinetics.

Emergency Checklist

❑ Closest staff desk or station

❑ Telephone

❑ Microphone

❑ Door alarms

❑ First-aid kit

❑ Water faucet

❑ Fire extinguisher

❑ Fire sprinkler placement

❑ Closest available wheelchair

❑ Emergency exit

From *Exercise for Frail Elders* by E. Best-Martini and K. A. Botenhagen-DiGenova, 2003, Champaign, IL: Human Kinetics.

The American Red Cross *First-Aid Manual* (2003) has a list of symptoms that require immediate professional medical attention:

- Unconsciousness
- Difficulty breathing
- Persistent chest pain or pressure
- Severe bleeding
- Seizures
- Severe headache
- Slurred speech
- Broken bones
- Spinal injuries

Along with caring for the individual in distress, make sure that the other participants are safe and remain calm. By staying calm yourself, you will keep your class members feeling confident and safe.

GOOD SENSATION AND BAD SENSATION OR PAIN

You need to be alert for any participant who experiences pain while exercising. Remind all participants to stop and tell you immediately if they feel any pain while exercising. Your observations and interventions help keep them injury free. In addition, you should observe and evaluate their exercise technique (see the section "Three-Step Instructional Process" in chapter 3) to determine whether their technique or position is causing the problem. Awareness of poor technique is important when teaching frail elders and adults with special needs. Use the motto "Train, don't strain."

It is common for people to associate pain with a negative experience. There is a difference between "good" sensation and "bad" sensation or pain when exercising. Good sensation is a sign that you are working out at the appropriate level. Table 2.1 describes types of sensation or pain and how to determine whether it is good or bad. The areas to evaluate are the location of the sensations, how it feels after exercising, and what it means.

If you determine that the sensation is bad pain, have the participant stop exercising immediately. Figure 2.1 shows some tips for responding to bad sensation or pain. For example, the exercise can be modified by decreasing the weight (if any), decreasing the number of repetitions, adjusting the speed of movement, adjusting the body position or mechanics of the movement, or replacing the exercise with one that feels better. See chapter 8 for more information on how to modify exercises. We recommend that you copy this figure for your participants to keep and review. They should discuss any bad sensations or pain with their physicians. Any new recommendations by the physician can be logged in the "modified goal" column of the Fitness Leader's Log form.

TABLE 2.1	GOOD SENSATION VERSUS BAD SENSATION OR PAIN

	Good sensation	Bad sensation or pain
Sensation	Dull soreness	Sharp pain
Location	In the muscle, not the joint	In or near the joint
Duration	Relieved within minutes after exercise	Continues to hurt after exercise
Next session	Less soreness with the same effort	No improvement or worsens
What it means	Normal muscle fatigue	Problem with a joint or muscle

From STRONG WOMEN STAY YOUNG by Miriam E. Nelson, PhD, and Sarah Wernick, PhD, copyright © 1997 by Miriam E. Nelson and Sarah Wernick. Used by permission of Bantam Books, a division of Random House, Inc.

From *Exercise for Frail Elders* by E. Best-Martini and K. A. Botenhagen-DiGenova, 2003, Champaign, IL: Human Kinetics.

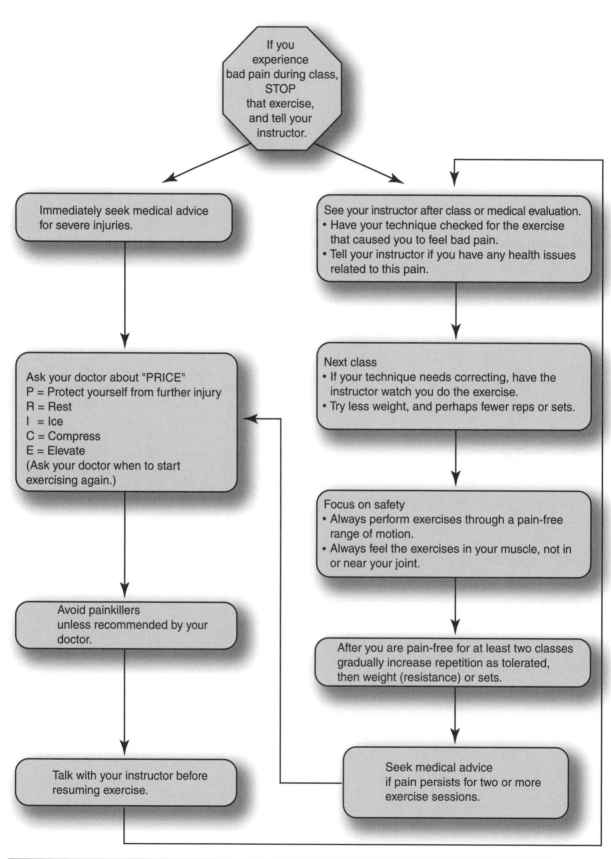

FIGURE 2.1 Tips for responding to bad sensation or pain.

From *Exercise for Frail Elders* by E. Best-Martini and K. A. Botenhagen-DiGenova, 2003, Champaign, IL: Human Kinetics.

Large-Group Safety Checklist

❑ With a large group, your need for good observation and communication skills increases. Safety becomes more difficult to ensure when you are unable to be totally attentive to all participants.

❑ Be prepared for new participants to join before you know their limitations and needs. Consider seating them next to you for the first few sessions.

❑ Keep all equipment and supplies within safe reach and in a safe location.

❑ Do not keep weights, if used, at each participant's place. Instead, keep them close to you on a cart, and distribute them when needed.

❑ You may limit the exercise class to just the warm-up session to make a larger group more manageable. This is described in chapters 4 and 8.

❑ When possible, create two smaller exercise groups instead of one large one.

❑ Find a co-leader to make two pairs of eyes available. You both may lead, or one can lead while the other spots participants.

❑ Review the room setup charts in chapter 3 (figures 3.1 and 3.2). They provide guidance for the physical setup of the room and the arrangement of participants and supplies. There are two seating variations, depending on the number of participants in the class. When you plan the room layout, remember to take into account the space needed for both wheelchairs and leg-extending foot pedals on the wheelchairs.

From *Exercise for Frail Elders* by E. Best-Martini and K. A. Botenhagen-DiGenova, 2003, Champaign, IL: Human Kinetics.

SAFETY IN LARGE GROUPS

Another area that can affect safety is how large the exercise class is. A group is considered large when it has so many students that you cannot watch each one do each exercise. The size of the exercise group depends on the location, instructor, and participants. A group may grow as enrollment in the facility grows. It is important that you have a strategy for teaching a large exercise group. See the large-group safety checklist for tips.

Motivation and safety help you create a successful exercise program. The final step is ensuring that the program is effective.

MAKE IT EFFECTIVE

An exercise program is effective when it focuses on function, fitness, and fun and meets the needs and goals of the individual participants. Effectiveness or an effective program design includes consideration of motivation (without motivation individuals will not come to class), safety (if an individual becomes injured, he or she will not be able to exercise), and the following:

- Realistic goals must be set by the participant and the leader in collaboration.

- The leader needs to observe and remain informed about each participant's current functional status.

- The exercise program should be based on professional fitness standards.

- The exercise class needs to adhere to safety guidelines.

- The exercise components (described in the next section) need to follow a structured sequence as reviewed in part II of this book.

Let's look more closely at the exercise components.

EFFECTIVE USE OF THE EXERCISE PROGRAM COMPONENTS

The components of the exercise programs that are offered in this book are

- warm-up exercises,
- aerobic exercises,
- resistance exercises, and
- cool-down exercises.

Each of these components is important and has specific goals and benefits.

1. Warm-up exercises ensure a smooth transition between the resting and exercising states. Warm-up includes posture, breathing, and range-of-motion exercises.

2. Aerobic exercises enhance cardiovascular endurance, usually by means of sustained large-muscle activity (e.g., walking, swimming, cycling, bicycling).

3. Resistance exercises strengthen all the major muscle groups. Balance exercises can be included to decrease the risk of falls.

4. Cool-down exercises ensure a smooth transition between the exercising and resting states. Cool-down includes stretching and flexibility exercises to increase flexibility in the major joints, particularly in injury-prone hip, trunk, and shoulder areas. Relaxation, stress-reduction, and breathing techniques can be included in this component or taught for use outside class.

Table 2.2 helps you understand the effective use of each component. Chapter 8 provides many options for combining the exercise components into an effective exercise program. For example, for beginners or as a buildup to resistance training, you may start by teaching only the warm-up component—gentle exercises that are easy to learn and appropriate for all participants. With the information in chapter 8, you will be able to customize comprehensive exercise programs.

EFFECTIVE EXERCISE PROGRAM DESIGN

For an exercise program to be effective, it must meet individual participants' needs and adhere to current standards of fitness programming for older adults. The U.S. Surgeon General recommends that

TABLE 2.2	COMPONENTS OF AN EXERCISE PROGRAM				
Component	Includes these exercises	Repetitions per exercise[a]	Duration of a single exercise or repetition	Duration per 45- to 60-minute class	Major benefits
Warm-up	• Range-of-motion • Low-intensity aerobics	4–8	2 seconds per repetition	10 minutes minimum	• Increases internal body temperature • Injury prevention
Aerobics	• Aerobic exercises (such as walking, swimming, cycling)	Varies	Varies[b]	15–30 minutes	• Cardiorespiratory endurance
Resistance Training	• Body-weight exercise[c] • Resistance exercises	8–15	6 seconds per repetition	15–30 minutes	• Muscular strength and endurance
Cool-down	• Stretching exercises[d]	1	15–30 seconds per stretch	5–30 minutes	• Improved flexibility
	• Relaxation techniques • Stress-reduction techniques	Varies	Varies	5–30 minutes	• Relaxation, stress reduction

[a]Several factors determine the number of repetitions, such as the component of exercise, the level of fitness of the participant, the level of progress for that exercise, day-to-day variations in the participant's physical state, and the total amount of time available for the exercise class.
[b]Varies according to the type and beat of the music.
[c]Body-weight exercises are exercises in which one's body weight, such as the weight of one's arms or legs, serves as the resistance.
[d]The cool-down from aerobics also includes range-of-motion and low-intensity aerobic exercises.

older adults engage in some form of moderate exercise most days of the week. Moderate exercise is defined as 30 minutes of calorie-burning activities, such as walking and stationary cycling, three to seven days a week. The exercises presented in part II of this book adhere to the U.S. Surgeon General's exercise guidelines and the standards set by the American College of Sports Medicine, the American Council on Exercise, the American Senior Fitness Association, the National Institute on Aging, and the YMCA of the USA. See chapters 4 through 7 for specific guidelines for warm-ups, aerobics, resistance training, and stretching exercises. Chapter 8 will help you put these exercise components together into an effective exercise program design. Table 2.3 summarizes the F.I.T. (*F* for frequency, *I* for intensity, and *T* for time) guidelines for aerobics, resistance training, and stretching.

We highly recommend that you know your participants' abilities and limitations and introduce exercise slowly. Start with one or two days a week if that is all they can physically or mentally tolerate. If participants cannot attend two exercise classes a week, suggest types of exercises they can try on their own (with their physician's approval). The ACSM (1998a) recommends that you use a gradual approach, perhaps doing just one type of exercise, with the long-term goal of adding other forms of exercise. As participants' strength and endurance increase, you can help them increase the frequency, intensity, time, and type of exercises. In addition, make the program one that people will want to be members of. If the experience is positive, if people are enjoying each other as much as the exercises, you have added the secret element of fun. The fun of physical activity is what brings people back to recreate the experience and encourages them to include physical activity in their lives on a regular basis.

SUMMARY

The frail elderly and adults with special needs benefit greatly from physical activity. They can show a greater response rate to exercise than more active older adults. This audience needs fitness leaders who are aware of motivational, safety, and professional standards for making their exercise successful and effective.

The first key to creating an exercise program is motivation. Motivation may come from intrinsic motivators such as losing weight or trying something new. It also may stem some from extrinsic goals such as pursuing advanced training or achieving an award. It is very important for fitness leaders to understand participants' intrinsic and extrinsic goals because these motivators keep participants coming back to an exercise class. Motivational strategies such as realistic goal setting keep participants motivated both intrinsically and extrinsically over time because participants see and feel changes in their function, mood, strength, and flexibility as they progress.

The second key to creating an exercise program is safety. As noted in this chapter, at any age, physical exercise carries risks. The exercise program is safe when it is designed with both the individual's and group's strengths and limitations in mind. Through a physician's medical clearance, a thorough fitness assessment, and your vigilant observations during

TABLE 2.3	EXERCISE PROGRAM DESIGN FOR OLDER ADULT F.I.T.NESS		
Exercise component	**Frequency**	**Intensity**	**Time**
Aerobics	3–5 days per week	12–14 on the RPE[a] scale ("somewhat hard")	20–30 continuous minutes of low to moderate work
Resistance training	2 to 3 times per week on nonconsecutive days when doing a full-body workout	Initially, perform 8–15 repetitions of a resistance exercise at an exertion level perceived as very light to light (an RPE of 9–11). Progress to "somewhat hard" (an RPE of 12–14) when appropriate, after excellent technique is learned.	Not applicable
Stretching	2 to 7 times per week	Stretches should be taken only to the point of tightness or mild intensity, not pain.	10–30 seconds per stretch, except 5 seconds or less for neck stretches

[a]RPE (Rating of Perceived Exertion) scale is a useful tool for monitoring exercise intensity (Borg 1998; see figure 5.1).

class you can ensure that participants are exercising at a level that is appropriate for them. Following established and recommended safety guidelines like those provided in this chapter as well as reviewing educational handouts and planning regular group discussions on safety topics will keep safety at the forefront of your exercise class.

The third key to creating an exercise class is effectiveness. An exercise program is effective when it meets the motivational and safety needs of participants mentioned above, but also meets certain professional standards. These professional standards include effective use of the exercise program components. The four main exercise components offered in this book are warm-up exercises, aerobic exercises, resistance exercises, and cool-down exer-

cises. Each of these components is important and has specific goals and benefits necessary for a well-rounded exercise program and follow guidelines from the U.S. Surgeon General and other leading organizations in the field of health and fitness such as the American College of Sports Medicine, the American Council on Exercise, the American Senior Fitness Association, and the National Institute on Aging.

The combination of motivation, safety, and effective program components helps you to create an exercise class that meets individual as well as group goals. A well-designed program promotes functional independence at all levels and is a fun and enjoyable experience.

CHAPTER 3

THE LEADER: STEPS TO SUCCESS

> "People must believe that leaders understand their needs and have their interests at heart. . . . Leaders breathe life into the hopes and dreams of others and enable them to see exciting possibilities that the future holds."
>
> *Kouzes and Posner 1995*

Frail elders and adults with special needs who participate in your exercise class look to you as the leader to exhibit the qualities expressed in the quote that opens this chapter. It is important for you to determine and conscientiously monitor what your participants need from you as their fitness leader.

This chapter discusses how to develop leadership skills and to incorporate leadership strategies in your exercise class. We share with you our own tips for positive leadership.

CREATING A SENSE OF FUN AND COMMUNITY

What activities do you look forward to attending? Most likely they are activities that are interactive, educational, and fun. You may look forward to going because of the instructor or the other participants. An interactive, educational, and fun atmosphere is what you want to instill in your class. The following sections present some strategies for creating a warm and welcoming environment, promoting common goals for the group, and encouraging friendships and social support.

CREATING A WARM AND WELCOMING ENVIRONMENT

As mentioned in chapter 2, participants join your group for different reasons. As you become more familiar with individual participants, you can begin to facilitate social interaction among them. As participants get to know one another, a sense of community begins to develop. Here are some ways to encourage a warm environment.

- Be organized and ready for your participants to arrive. This gives them the message that you are eagerly awaiting their arrival.
- Have everyone wear name tags during class to learn each other's names.
- Be sure that participants feel welcome. Know each individual's name, and welcome participants by name. Ask what they prefer to be called. Never assume that elderly people prefer to be called by their first name.
- Avoid using terms such as "sweetie," "honey," or "guys." These terms can make participants feel uncomfortable and insulted.
- As a group, choose a name for your exercise class.
- Create a display board describing the exercise class. It can include photos of participants along with group goals and reminders.
- Have the class create new names for the exercises in part II. Names that your class originates can be easier for participants to remember. It also helps them feel that this is their class, which is a good motivator.

- Put the group's name on exercise supply items. The name can be painted on exercise towels, vests, T-shirts, or hats. This reinforces a sense of teamwork.
- Keep an attendance chart on a large board to graphically show the attendance and progress of participants. This board can be a visual motivator for participants.
- Acknowledge individual successes. You can show physical progress through a photo timeline.
- Help participants feel the fun of physical activity. Be sure to laugh, and encourage a sense of playfulness. Be sure that no participant misinterprets your laughter as ridicule.

PROMOTING GROUP GOALS

First help each participant in your class identify his or her individual goal(s) (see the section "Goal Setting" in chapter 2). Having common goals as a group helps to create a sense of fun and community. They are group goals because they are created together with all members and leaders. The same focus on realistic and obtainable goals that apply to individual goals also apply to group goals.

Here are some ideas for group goals:

- To feel welcome
- To know the names of other participants
- To see personal progress through attendance records and photos
- To be aware of posture and positioning
- To be able to identify the muscles targeted by specific exercises
- To describe the muscles involved in the exercises
- To build endurance and muscular strength
- To have fun and feel part of something special
- To present the exercises to other groups
- To understand the physiological and psychological benefits of physical activity (see appendixes A and B)

ENCOURAGING FRIENDSHIPS AND SOCIAL SUPPORT

Many of your participants may live in settings other than their own private homes. Previous relationships with family and friends may have been altered by this relocation. Recreation and wellness programs can promote a sense of culture and community that help people once again feel part of a social network. Social activity and friendships help people stay well as much as physical activity through exercise does. The importance of adult friendship was researched by Rosemary Blieszner and Rebecca G. Adams. One of their findings was that "good friends are critically important to successful aging. . . . Friends can be more important to the psychological well being of older adults than even family members are" (Blieszner and Adams 1992, 112). You can help create feelings of ease, warmth, and friendship within the exercise group. Be sure that your room is set up before the class so that participants come into a welcoming environment. Advance preparation helps create a friendly setting where people feel safe and comfortable.

New friends are perhaps one of the most important contributions that you can offer participants. You can encourage friendships and nurture a sense of community within the group in subtle ways. Here are some ideas:

- Once you are familiar with the group, seat individuals next to one another for specific reasons. For example, a gregarious person can be encouraging to another who is less confident. A new participant can be seated next to the leader to be introduced to the group.
- Use exercises and activities that encourage participants to look at one another, such as an initial "hello" to the person seated next to them or tossing a balloon while calling out the name of the intended catcher.
- Promote socialization and friendship within your group. Participants are interested in each other's lives and experiences. For participants with communication losses who cannot share their stories with others, if you know about participants' lives, you can ask whether they would like for you to share their stories.
- Acknowledge the absence of any member. Other participants wonder and worry why someone is missing, even though they may not verbalize their concern. Remember that confidentiality is of great importance. Check with the staff and the participant in question before sharing personal information about him or her.
- Always be honest so that participants can learn to trust you.
- Be compassionate. If a participant is in the hospital, you could bring a get-well card to

class for others to sign. Your concern gives participants the message that they are part of a community of caring individuals.

- Depending on the size of your group, you may want to celebrate birthdays. You can also celebrate other occasions, such as holidays and exercise accomplishments.

How to Set Up a Group Exercise Class

Your responsibilities as a fitness leader begin before the actual class takes place. The following sections offer some tips for successfully preparing for your class and some important issues to consider before teaching frail elderly participants and adults with special needs. After reviewing the setup, you should consider the organization and use of supplies and equipment. The final section can help you decide whether to use music in your class.

Preparing to Work With the Participants

There are many factors to consider before you officially greet the participants and open the class. A new fitness leader needs to consider some of the issues that he or she may encounter while working with participants who are frail or have special needs. Best Martini, Weeks, and Wirth (2003) list some common challenges that require understanding and sensitivity from the leader:

Passivity	Hyperactivity
Anxiety	Confusion
Lack of response	Embarrassment

Tips for Preparing for Class

❑ Identify good candidates for participation in the class.

❑ Request physician's approval or physician's orders for each participant. A sample form for this purpose appears in appendix C. The staff, the participant, and family members can assist you in filling out the cover letter and form to submit for the physician's approval and signature. Review the physician's recommendations with the participant. See chapter 2 for more details.

❑ Send an approval notice to the participant's family or responsible party if the participant is not living at home.

❑ Establish individual goals with each participant (see chapter 2).

❑ Keep a binder containing the medical clearance forms and Fitness Leader's Log (in chapter 2) for all participants.

❑ Be familiar with specific recommendations and issues identified by the physician on the medical clearance form.

❑ Depending on the setting of your class, let the appropriate staff members know who will attend and what time the class starts. Some of your participants may need assistance with personal care or transportation before class.

❑ Remind participants (and any staff members who help them dress) to dress casually and wear athletic shoes or walking shoes.

❑ Have your attendance displays and informational materials ready for use.

From *Exercise for Frail Elders* by E. Best-Martini and K. A. Botenhagen-DiGenova, 2003, Champaign, IL: Human Kinetics..

Loneliness

Low self-esteem

Feelings of uselessness

Dependency

Cognitive losses

Short attention span

Lack of purpose

Sensory losses

Depression

Anger

Wandering

You may need to address one or more of these issues in your class, depending on the setting and the number of participants. Each of these challenges requires a response in either your attitude or your action as the leader. Your sensitivity will help you to determine the best response. Suppose that you are beginning a new exercise in your class. Five participants are not moving or responding to your verbal and physical cues. Before you jump to the conclusion that your teaching style is weak, look more closely at these individuals. They may not be re-

sponding because they are embarrassed, are passive by nature, are depressed, have low self-esteem, or have visual and auditory losses. There are many reasons for lack of participation. Get to know your individual participants and you will be able to help them become more active and feel better about themselves.

Now you are ready to learn how to prepare the physical environment, supplies, and equipment for the exercise class.

SETTING UP THE ROOM AND SUPPLIES

The physical environment of your class needs to be looked at closely. A good room arrangement can enhance interaction between the participants and the fitness leader. We recommend that you create a chart of your room layout. Room setup varies with the size of the group. Figures 3.1 and

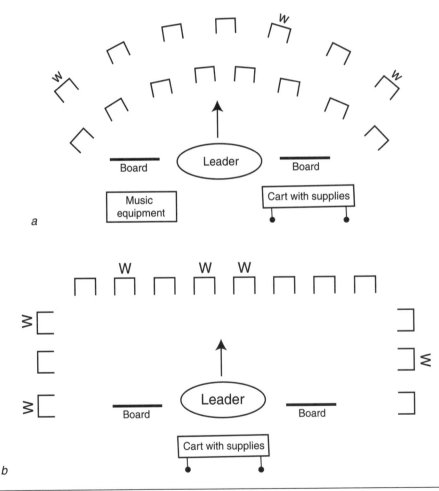

a

b

FIGURE 3.1 Room setup for 15 or fewer participants: *(a)* semicircle and *(b)* open box.

3.2 show different room setups. Figure 3.1 shows two schemes—the semicircle and open box—for setting up for a group of 15 or fewer participants; the chart in figure 3.2 is for more than 15 participants. We highly recommend an assistant or co-instructor for larger groups. We also offer a checklist for further help in preparing your class site.

The list of equipment in appendix I offers ideas about the supplies and equipment that can work well for your group. As you add to your collection of exercise equipment and supplies, we recommend the purchase of a cart with wheels to store and transport them.

Resistance bands and tubes—stretchy, rubber-band-like devices—are inexpensive and safe resistance-training tools. However, exercises that use these devices can be more challenging for the instructor to explain and demonstrate and for the participants to perform than exercises that use free weights. Resistance bands and tubes can be tied to wheelchair arms or bed rails for push-and-pull exercises. Bands and tubes come in at least three different resistances—light, medium, and heavy—and can be doubled up to increase the workload. Sponges of various sizes and shapes can be used to squeeze and grip for improving hand strength.

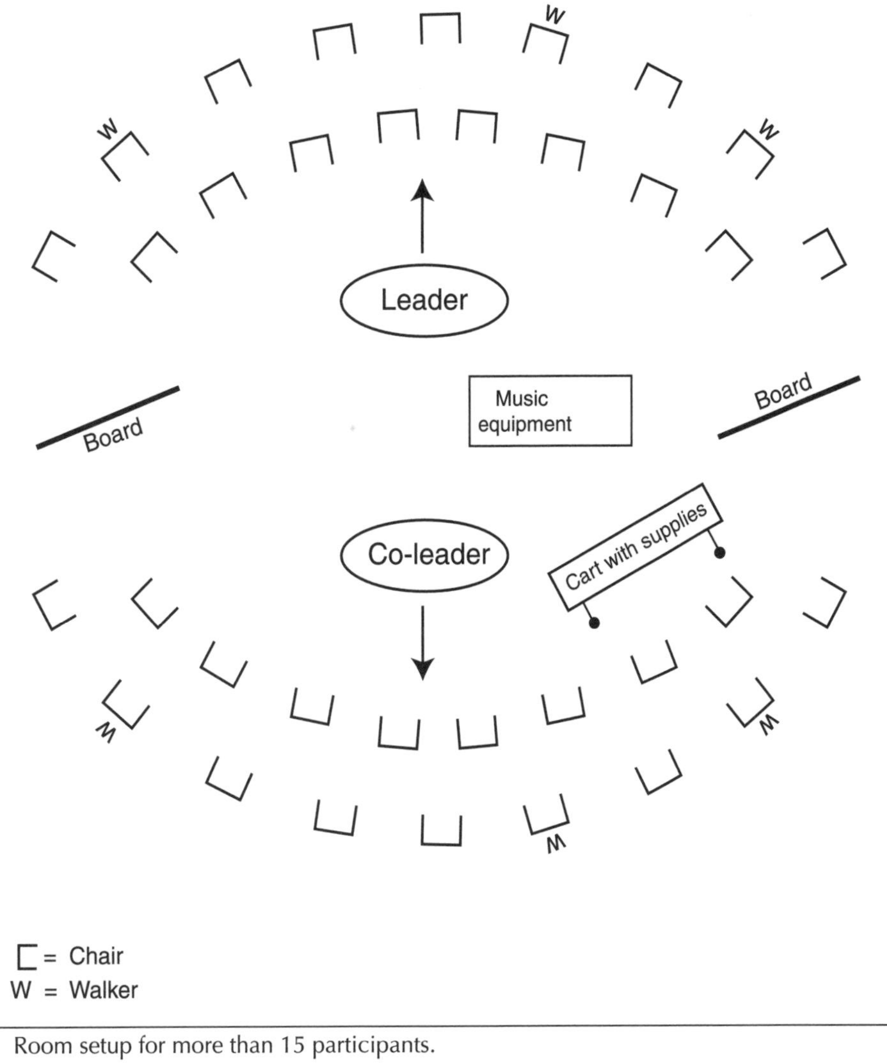

FIGURE 3.2   Room setup for more than 15 participants.

Checklist for Setting Up the Furniture, Equipment, and Supplies

Furniture

❏ Have the room set up before participants arrive.

❏ Arrange chairs, and remember to allow space for wheelchairs within the circle.

❏ Determine whether the chairs should have arms or no arms. This is an important consideration for proper exercise technique and individual safety needs. It is easier to do exercises in chairs without arms. However, participants with balance problems who are at high risk of falls may feel more secure in chairs with arms. Most fitness leaders need to be flexible and make do with the chairs that are available at the class site. Keep in mind that some of your participants will probably be seated in wheelchairs.

❏ Arrange the furniture so that participants are not looking into the sun or glare. Their backs should be to the window or light whenever possible.

❏ Arrange the furniture so that all participants can focus on the leader. You can sit in the middle of a circle, a semicircle, an open box group setup diagram (as described in figures 3.1 and 3.2), or double circles, depending on the size of the group.

Equipment and Supplies

❏ Find a corner or other out-of-the-way location to store any walkers. Many participants feel more secure knowing that their walkers are directly behind their chairs. A walker with brakes can make a good prop for some of the exercises; for example, it can facilitate the transition from sitting to standing.

❏ If you decide to use music, have the tape deck or CD player close by so that you can change the music or lower the sound when needed. A sound system may already be set up at the site so that you do not need to bring your own equipment.

❏ Eliminate competing sights and sounds. If there is a television in the room, be sure that both the sound and the picture are turned off.

❏ Set up all of your visual props. These may include a poster of muscles, attendance records, name of the group, inspirational pictures, or the exercise routine in large print. They should be displayed in an uncluttered way. You can vary the visual props according to seasonal themes or the type of exercises that will be done.

❏ Focusing on an object at about eye level is a good technique for promoting balance. You can put a mark or line on the wall at a height of about 5 feet 2 inches to 5 feet 7 inches (1.6 to 1.7 meters) for those who stand while exercising. You can display a beautiful poster or picture for participants to focus on instead of a bare wall. These visual aids can also be used in the relaxation and visualization exercises found in chapter 7.

❏ Make a copy of the exercises in part II. These can be placed on a clipboard for your reference while teaching.

❏ Keep exercise supplies and equipment in a convenient location so that you can pass them out safely and quickly when needed. Appendix I describes various types of equipment that can enhance your class.

❏ Place exercise equipment in a safe place not readily accessible to participants who could injure themselves by misusing it. You need to control the use of weights to ensure safety.

From *Exercise for Frail Elders* by E. Best-Martini and K. A. Botenhagen-DiGenova, 2003, Champaign, IL: Human Kinetics.

Vinyl-covered dumbbells are color-coded for easy identification by weight. The vinyl-coated weights can be less intimidating than traditional metal dumbbells, especially for beginners. You can use these colors to encourage participants' progress. For example, one possibility is to award a red ribbon for mastering a red weight. Be creative.

When your budget does not allow for conventional resistance-training equipment, you can make your own weights, such as a sock or glove filled with rice or sand. A long tube sock works best (knot the open end or tie the two ends together). Refer to appendix I for more creative ideas.

The physical therapy department or medical supply office of your facility may be able to recommend additional resistance-training products and distributors. Find out whether your medical supply office can order soft surgical tubing, which can be cut into 3-foot (0.9-meter) lengths and tied at the ends to form resistance tubes for push-pull exercises. Sometimes the facility or instructor purchases the equipment, sometimes participants pay for their own.

Tips for Deciding Whether to Use Music

Another important issue to consider is whether to use music during the exercise class. Music is optional. The decision to use music or not will be up to you as the fitness leader. Remember, safety and participant success should always come first in making this decision. Ask your participants whether they would like music during the class. If you decide to use music, ask the participants for their favorite types of music. This helps create a sense of community within your group.

These are some advantages of using music:

- Music creates a welcoming environment.
- Music sets the mood.
- Music motivates and energizes participants.
- Music might be used during certain parts of the program but not others.
- Music awakens the spirit and energizes participants with extreme limitations of movement. Even if they can move only their toes or fingers, they can tap along with the music.
- Music adds variety to the exercise class.
- Music of a specific type fosters camaraderie among the individuals who helped select it.

These are some disadvantages of using music:

- Music can be a distraction and can decrease attention span.
- Music can drown out your instructions to participants.
- Participants with hearing losses may find the music irritating when it is too loud or the pitch is too high.
- Some music can overstimulate participants who are trying to follow directions.
- Participants have different individual and cultural tastes in music. The music one person may love to exercise to, another may dislike.

If you decide to use music, we offer the following tips:

- You can play soft music or sounds of nature to welcome participants and begin the warm-up.
- Be sure that whatever type of music you use is in sync with the specific exercises. For example, music played during the welcome should be soft and inviting. The warm-up should have music with sustained, flowing sounds that encourage participants to take their time in their movements and to be aware of their breathing and posture. The aerobic component can use lively, faster-paced music. You might not play any music during the resistance-training component so that everyone can focus on counting and form. The cooldown should have relaxing music that again promotes slower movements.
- Many older adults favor music that was popular when they were in their teens and twenties for long-term reminiscing. However, people who have grown up with music continue to appreciate and listen to new sounds. Do not limit yourself or your participants. If you decide to use music, take the opportunity to introduce new types of music so that participants feel more a part of today's world.
- You always consider what the majority of participants want and enjoy.

Because of the variety of individual tastes, we do not want to recommend specific musical tapes. However, in the recommended resources, we list some companies that you can contact for good exercise musical tapes.

Helpful Tips for Opening Your Exercise Class

Each session should begin with a welcome and a description of the upcoming exercise routine to give structure to the class. After the welcome, tell the participants what is to be covered in the class. This review can help alleviate participants' anxiety regarding exercising. Remind the group about the importance of safety. Safety comes first in all aspects of the exercise program. You can also use this time to educate participants about exercise, health, healthy lifestyles, prevention, and wellness. The following sections look at the welcome, safety, and education in more detail.

The Welcome

The welcome sets the tone for your class. This is where the stage is set for all group work. In addition to establishing rapport with your group, you can also use this time to observe each member and to detect individual needs.

Tips for the Welcome

- Always start the class with a welcome. You can greet each person individually by name and shake his or her hand. While welcoming each person, you can ask how he or she is feeling that day.
- While you are greeting participants, really observe each person. Are they responsive to your greeting? Do they have their hearing aids on?
- Are there any new participants whom you have not met yet? Do they have medical clearance to participate?
- Does anyone appear to be sleepier than usual? Does anyone appear to have a change in mood or attitude? These are all possible signs of emotional stress, new medications, or overmedication. They also are possible indicators of a change in medical status. Be very observant.
- Open the class with a friendly greeting, such as, "Welcome to our exercise class. I am so happy to see each of you here today."
- You can begin the class by announcing the day's inspirational or fitness theme or simply the date.

Physiological and emotional changes frequently go unnoticed by those who work with frail elders and adults with special needs. Your observations can make all the difference in avoiding an emergency. This brings us to the importance of safety.

Focus on Safety

Safety is the cornerstone of any good exercise program. Every aspect of your work is based on a clear understanding of safety issues. Your role as leader is to instill this focus on safety in your participants. While you have everyone's attention during the welcoming phase of the class, use this opportunity to remind them about safety during the class.

Safety Tips

- Remind participants about the importance of good posture.
- Remind participants to follow you closely to ensure that they are using proper exercise techniques.
- Remind participants to breathe continuously during all exercises.
- Remind participants to immediately cease exercise if they experience any pain.
- Remind participants who need assistance with getting in and out of a chair to ask for help before getting up.
- Remind participants to go at their own pace and not to feel that they need to compete with others.
- Remind participants to be aware of one another while exercising in a close space.
- Remind participants to put exercise equipment and supplies in a safe location so that no one will trip over them.

Safety is important both within and outside the class. Your goal is to emphasize the importance of everyday safety to participants. Outside class, there are safety concerns related to walking, transferring from a chair to a walker, navigating steps and stairs, and eliminating fall risks in the home environment. Refer to chapter 2 for a review of general exercise safety guidelines.

FOCUS ON EDUCATION

Participants need to fully understand the role that they play in improving their strength, function, and independence. This understanding is created through education.

Education affects individual behaviors and builds the motivation that is needed to change a sedentary lifestyle. By seeing improvements in physical endurance and strength, participants can begin to see themselves as active and vital people. Their lifestyles and attitudes can improve dramatically. This personal perspective is extremely important for you to take into account.

We recommend that you provide information about fitness, *wellness* (the constant, deliberate effort to stay healthy physically and emotionally to achieve the highest potential for well-being), and healthy lifestyles issues during the exercise class. Some instructors use the end of the class for this information. You might want to cover specific topics over several classes. Add time for this to your class outline. The welcome and opening section or cool-down and closing section of the class are good opportunities to educate participants.

Table 3.1 offers some educational topics that you can address. We have included useful and informative material throughout the book that can be used as handouts, including these.

- Figure 1.1 Frailty
- Table 1.1 Common Medical Disorders
- Table 2.1 Good Sensation Versus Bad Sensation or Pain
- Figure 2.1 Tips for Responding to Bad Sensation or Pain
- Table 5.2 General Aerobic-Training Guidelines for Older Adults
- Table 6.1 Common Myths and Facts About Resistance Training
- Table 6.2 General Resistance-Training Guidelines for Older Adults
- Table 7.2 General Stretching Guidelines
- Appendix J Muscles of the Human Body

Many participants will take educational handouts with them and review them further. These handouts reinforce the information that you discuss during the exercise class.

TABLE 3.1	**EDUCATIONAL TOPICS FOR FITNESS AND WELLNESS**
Topic	**Activity**
Diet and nutrition	During the class, take a break to drink water. During the break, discuss the importance of diet and hydration.
Stress	While leading the stretching portion of the exercise program, discuss the benefits of relaxation and how it helps decrease stress and anxiety. Refer to chapter 4 (the sections on deep two-part breathing) and chapter 7 for more information. Remind participants to breathe deeply for stress reduction. Bring an inspirational quote to each class.
Social support	Friendship and social support are important issues to address. Encourage participants to get to know one another so that they can feel comfortable talking about personal issues with one another outside of class.
Physiological and psychological benefits of exercise	Use appendixes A and B to reinforce instruction about the benefits of exercise.
Healthy lifestyles	Have a theme for each class, such as staying active mentally and physically, sleeping well, making the home environment safer.
Muscle anatomy	Have participants get to know all the muscle groups that the exercises work. Appendix J offers a visual aid for you and your participants.

Successful Strategies for Leading Your Exercise Class

We want to present some strategies that can help you successfully lead a class for frail elders and adults with special needs. The three-step instructional process (table 3.2) gives you a structure in which to teach exercises safely and effectively. This technique is a foundation; later in this chapter we present specific strategies for teaching participants with communication, cognitive, and sensory losses.

Three-Step Instructional Process

The three-step instructional process helps you to lead exercise for frail elders and adults with special needs safely and effectively. In step 1 you demonstrate and describe each exercise. In step 2 you observe and evaluate your participants as they follow your lead. In step 3 you give your participants constructive, positive *feedback* (verbal or nonverbal instruction, assistance, and recommendations) as they continue to follow your lead. Feedback (step 3) can also be given between exercises. Steps 1 through 3 flow naturally together.

Step 1: Demonstrate and Describe

Describe how to do the exercise as you demonstrate it. Choose words that enable your participants to feel successful. For example, "Move your elbows toward each other," instead of "Move your elbows *together*." Questions can be an effective way to describe how to do the exercise; for example, "How close can you comfortably move your elbows toward each other?" Keep your instruction positive and encouraging: "The farther apart your elbows are from touching, the more potential you have for improvement." "Notice how your elbows get closer over time."

Demonstrate every exercise with proper technique and speed. Avoid the temptation to do a speedy demonstration. Remember, you are *modeling* the exercise (showing how to perform it). If any of your participants have trouble following you, demonstrate the exercise without words, not even counting. Always keep those participants dealing with visual impairments as close to you, the leader, as possible. Pay attention to how your participants learn best.

In beginning classes and for new participants or individuals with poor *carryover skills* (being able to apply or carry over techniques previously learned), such as those with memory loss, follow these ABCs to demonstrate and describe exercises:

• **A**ction. Briefly describe and demonstrate the *exercise technique:* the start position, highlights of the movement phase, and finish position, which is always the same as the start position. The start/finish position and highlights of the movement phase are referred to as the *critical checkpoints*. The critical checkpoints are described or illustrated for the exercises in chapters 4 through 7. The arrows in the photographs of these chapters indicate the direction of movement for each exercise.

• **B**reathing and other safety tips. Briefly describe *safety tips* as you continue demonstrating. Review the general safety guidelines in chapter 2. Specific safety tips for each exercise are given in chapters 4 through 7. Two important safety criteria are correct posture and breathing. Teach good posture and proper breathing, particularly not holding one's breath. Your participants cannot hold their breath if they are counting aloud. Therefore, have your participants count aloud, especially in beginning classes and large groups where it is not possible for you to check each participant's breathing.

• **C**ounting. Demonstrate the exercise about two more times as you *count aloud*. Counting varies with different types of exercise. Table 3.3 summarizes how and why to count with warm-ups, resistance training, aerobics, and stretching exercises. It is most important for partici-

Table 3.2	Three-Step Instructional Process

Step 1. Demonstrate and describe the ABCs of each exercise.
a. *A*ction
b. *B*reathing and other safety tips
c. *C*ounting

Step 2. Observe and evaluate (SEE each participant)
a. *S*afety precautions
b. *E*xercise technique
c. *E*ach individual's needs

Step 3. Give group and individual feedback.
a. Verbal
b. Visual nonverbal
c. Physical nonverbal

TABLE 3.3   HOW COUNTING VARIES AMONG THE DIFFERENT COMPONENTS OF EXERCISE

Components	Repetitions	How to count[a]	Why count
Warm-up	4–8	"1, and, 2, and, 3, and . . ." "1, and" = 1 repetition = 2 seconds	For slow and smooth pacing
Aerobics	1 or more	Varies according to the type and beat of the music.	To get and keep the pace
Resistance training	8–15	"1,1,1, up 1,1,1, down, 2,2,2, up, . . ." (or out and in instead of up and down.) "1,1,1, up" = 1 repetition = about 6–8 seconds	For slow and smooth pacing To ensure that participants are not holding their breath
Stretching	1	Count silently or visually with the second hand of a clock. Stretches are held 10–30 seconds (the same count on each side), except neck stretches, which are held only 5 seconds per side.	To start and stop the stretch

[a]First announce the number of repetitions of each exercise. Then count the repetitions of each exercise aloud, except for stretching.

pants to count aloud during resistance exercises because breath holding during these exercises presents a higher risk of increasing a participant's blood pressure. If participants are counting aloud, you know they cannot be holding their breath. Counting keeps participants engaged and can create a lively atmosphere. Count in the dominant language of the group, or have the participants take turns counting in their primary language.

After participants become familiar with the pace of the exercises by counting, instruct them to focus on their breathing instead of counting. If participants get off rhythm, recommend that they resume counting aloud. Remind your participants to count if you regularly have new participants or lead a large group without an assistant.

You will develop your own style of counting for each exercise component. For instance, you can look at the second hand of a clock to time a stretching exercise rather than counting aloud for a quieter, more relaxing atmosphere. Do what works best for you and your participants.

During step 2, observing and evaluating, counting can be a distraction for the instructor. However, you should count aloud initially to get the partici-

pants started. If the participants' counting fades during the exercise or if you notice anyone not counting, resume counting aloud with the participants.

If you do not have new participants in your class, you might use less demonstration and description of the exercises as your participants become more experienced. When they know the exercises, try skipping step 1. At that time, you can use just steps 2 and 3. However, individuals with poor carryover skills need at least a short demonstration and description of the exercises at every class.

STEP 2: OBSERVE AND EVALUATE

After a demonstration and description of the exercise (step 1), have participants follow you in performing the exercise. Observe and evaluate each participant. When observing and evaluating, pay attention to these areas, which you can remember by the acronym *SEE*:

Safety precautions — Observe general and specific safety guidelines for each exercise.

Exercise technique — Observe critical checkpoints.

Each individual's needs

Observe how this exercise addresses each participant's health needs and fitness goals.

Your class's performance determines the need for further cueing. No two classes are the same. You may have time to evaluate only the first two areas, especially if you are a new instructor or your participants are beginner exercisers. As you become more comfortable teaching the exercises and your participants become more experienced, you can begin to consider each individual's needs in your evaluation. Do your best to make time at the beginning of class to find out how your participants are feeling and at the end of class to find out how they responded to the exercises. If possible, let them know other times when you are available to discuss questions or concerns.

STEP 3: PROVIDE FEEDBACK

After your observation and evaluation of the class, as participants continue the exercise to its completion, give your participants feedback based on your observation and evaluation. The three types of feedback are verbal, visual nonverbal, and physical nonverbal.

Verbal Feedback   Keep your verbal feedback clear, concise, and positive. Be specific. Here are some examples of verbal feedback:

- Remind participants to count and not to hold their breath: "Mr. Judd, remember to count with us so we all keep the same pace."

- Ask pertinent questions to inspire active participation: "Does anyone know what leg muscle helps us get up out of a chair? The quadriceps helps us get up, and that is why the leg march exercise is so important."

- Acknowledge what they are doing well (individually or as a group): "Look at how much farther Mr. Judd can move through this exercise. What an improvement! Good work!" "Remember when we had a hard time completing 15 minutes of exercise? Now we are exercising for more than an hour. This is great progress!"

- Adjust the pace or rhythm: "Let's slow down our pace as we get ready to start our stretches."

- Motivate your participants to perform their best: "Let's look at this attendance board. It shows us how long we have been exercising together. It also shows us that each of you has progressed from 1-pound weights to 3- and 5-pound weights. Fantastic!"

Visual Nonverbal Feedback   When giving visual nonverbal cues, make sure all of your participants can see you. Here are some examples of visual nonverbal feedback:

- Demonstrate further from a different position.

- Show illustrations, such as a muscle anatomy chart.

- Speed up or slow down your own performance to adjust the pace or rhythm.

- Motivate your participants to perform their best by gestures such as clapping or a thumbs-up.

Physical Nonverbal Feedback   When giving physical nonverbal cues, remember to touch a participant only after he or she has given you permission. Here are some examples of physical nonverbal feedback:

- Gently assist a participant through the exercise. (Try using verbal or visual nonverbal cues first.)

- Adjust equipment.

- Motivate your participants to perform their best by physical acknowledgments such as a pat on the back.

You can also give feedback between exercises. Beginning classes need more feedback between exercises as participants learn safety precautions and proper exercise technique. The pace of the class is slower, which helps prevent overexertion. As your participants become more experienced, minimize feedback between exercises to maximize exercise time. Ultimately, you can flow gracefully from one exercise to the next.

It is appropriate for you to interrupt your leading of the exercise to give participants feedback when the benefits of assisting individual participants outweigh the benefits of remaining in front of the class. Use your best judgment. As your participants learn exercises, they benefit greatly from one-on-one attention. If you have an assistant or co-leader, you have more opportunity to help your participants individually.

Leadership can be seen as a dialogue. For this dialogue to take place, people must be able to understand and respond to each other, which requires listening well and the ability to understand and interpret the words spoken. This dialogue becomes a challenge if any of the participants are dealing with communication losses, cognitive losses, or sensory losses. For participants with these losses, nonverbal descriptions and dialogue become as important or more important than verbal descriptions and dialogue. Both your verbal and nonverbal communication skills need to be direct and clear to the participant. Let's look at strategies for teaching participants with communication, cognitive, and sensory losses.

STRATEGIES FOR TEACHING PARTICIPANTS WITH COMMUNICATION LOSSES

Participants who have communication losses, such as aphasia, require both verbal and nonverbal cues from the leader. They may understand but not be able to express their thoughts (expressive aphasia), or they may not be able to understand or interpret information (receptive aphasia). Some participants may experience both receptive and expressive aphasia (global aphasia). Such participants comprehend best with a multisensory approach. For a multisensory approach, you need to use visual and tactile aides to clarify directions and to provide physical, visual, and verbal cuing. Nonverbal and multisensory approaches help participants understand and learn better. Here are some communication strategies to incorporate into your leadership style.

- Keep good eye contact with the participants. They need to see your demonstration and hear your directions.
- Repeat directions and information.
- Add nonverbal cues.
- Use your facial expressions and positive nods of your head to reinforce a job well done.
- Treat each participant as an intelligent person.
- Participants dealing with communication losses may look closely for visual cues and reinforcers. Be sure that you are a good model for them. Look professional, and always wear athletic shoes and appropriate attire. Avoid too many contrasting colors in your outfits. It may be difficult to see you and your cues if your outfit is too busy-looking.
- Give the participant time to respond to you. It may take them a little longer.
- Avoid too many distractions in the surrounding environment while you are trying to communicate. Extraneous noises and activity can decrease participants' comprehension.

- Avoid any language or form of communication that may seem demeaning to the participant.
- Speak to participants as you would to a friend in conversation.

STRATEGIES FOR TEACHING PARTICIPANTS WITH COGNITIVE LOSSES

Every setting where there are frail elders and adults with special needs includes someone who has some *cognitive loss* (an inability to perform normal cognitive functions, such as judgment, problem solving, communication, interpretation of environmental stimuli, memory, abstract thought, and paying attention). People with cognitive losses respond well to multisensory instruction as the *sensory* memory is the most intact.

Here are some leadership strategies for teaching participants with cognitive losses:

- Treat each participant as an intelligent person. Cognition is only a small part of who we are. People with cognitive losses still have many skills and talents.
- Smile and help all participants feel welcome.
- Keep your directions simple.
- Slow down your conversation and also the tempo of the exercises.
- Make good eye contact, and remember that nonverbal cues work well.
- Use many colorful visual props. They add the element of fun which helps to reduce any anxiety regarding their ability to understand directions in addition to encouraging attention.
- Repetition reinforces learning and is a very successful strategy when working with people with any level of memory loss.
- Provide structure and routine in each session. This continuity helps participants retain information.
- Allow extra time for participants with cognitive losses to respond to questions or directions. It may take them longer.
- Keep the environment as uncluttered and quiet as possible to keep it from being over-stimulating.
- Give a lot of positive feedback to participants.
- Provide cuing when needed.

- Break down instructions and exercises into smaller steps to make them easier to understand and follow. This strategy is called *task segmentation*. The steps are then added together to perform the complete task. Task segmentation can be used to teach new skills or forgotten skills.

- Be aware that many participants can no longer retain a learned skill from class to class. You may need to teach the same skills and exercises repeatedly, because they may seem new to some individuals with cognitive losses.

- Remember that participants with cognitive losses want to communicate normally and feel frustrated when they struggle with words.

The cuing strategies in table 3.4 have proven successful in teaching participants with cognitive losses. Table 3.4 also provides some examples of implementing these strategies.

Strategies for Teaching Participants With Sensory Losses

Some of your participants may have sensory losses. In addition to normal physiologic changes of aging, many elderly people experience a loss of one or more of the five senses (sight, hearing, taste, touch, and smell). The most noticeable sensory losses affect sight and hearing. However, less obvious sensory losses are still significant. A participant may have a loss of sensation in the hands and feet. This is important for you to know about. An individual with a sensory loss may feel very removed from the experience enjoyed by other participants. Participants with sensory losses need clear directions and visual or auditory reinforcements. Here are some leadership strategies for teaching participants with sensory losses:

- Use gestures and physical examples of what you verbally describe. The gestures need to be dramatic to emphasize the directions. The gestures can include facial expressions.

- Always check to be sure that participants are wearing their glasses or hearing aides.

- Seat participants with visual or hearing losses nearest you.

- Show large illustrations of specific exercises as a visual aid. The illustrations of specific exercises found in chapters 4 through 7 can be enlarged for this purpose.

- Provide exercise props that help reinforce the movements and techniques. Scarves and resistance bands help reinforce movements. Scarves are also colorful sensory enhancers. Pinwheels can be used during breathing exercises to help participants see their breath at work.

TABLE 3.4	Cuing Strategies for Teaching Participants With Cognitive Losses
Cuing technique	**Example**
Visual demonstration	Demonstrate the exercise for the participant. Look directly at the participant and speak clearly and simply. Be sure that you make eye contact and encourage the participant to "mirror" or copy your movements with him or her. Perform the visual demonstration very slowly.
Verbal prompts	Clearly state to the participant how to do the exercise: "Mr. Williams, move your fingers as if you are playing the piano."
Physical prompts	Physically initiate the movement for the participant. Always ask permission before physically touching a participant: "Mr. Williams, may I help lift your arms to get you started?"
Physical assistance	Physically assist the participant with the exercise. This type of cueing helps move the participant through the exercise even if he or she is unable to perform it alone. This step is a *hand over hand* movement with the leader assisting the participant with her or his hands. "Mr. Williams, look how we are playing the piano together hand in hand." Always ask permission before physically touching a participant.
Feedback	Give immediate feedback and reinforcement for the exercise and interaction. "Well done, Mr. Williams. Thank you for participating with me."

Adapted, by permission, from R.P. Katsinas, 1995, Excess disability. Presented at American Therapeutic Recreation Society Conference, Louisville, KY.

- Write the names of the muscles and the exercise on a large board. Have participants read and repeat them to reinforce the information.
- The loss of sensation (touch) can leave participants unaware of a region of their bodies, so always be sure to focus on the area that is moving, such as a leg, an arm, or the fingers. Encourage participants to touch this part to enhance body awareness and circulation.

HELPFUL TIPS FOR CLOSING YOUR EXERCISE CLASS

The closure of the class is as important as the opening and welcome. Just as you began the class with a warm welcome and acknowledgment of individual participants, you address some closing remarks to the group and some to each participant individually. After the participants have said good-bye and the class is formally over, you still have some finishing touches to complete.

THE CLOSING

The closing of the group should be integrated naturally into the framework of the exercise class. The final component of an exercise class, the cool-down, is intended to slow down the pace, stretch the muscles, and encourage participants to relax. While cooling down and encouraging relaxation, your voice should soften but still be audible to those hard of hearing. Some participants may be looking forward to the end of the class, while others wish that the group could stay together longer. Remember that some of your participants are here for the social and emotional connections rather than physical exercise. You should establish a clear signal that the class is about to end. This signal is important to provide structure, especially for participants with sensory or cognitive losses. Here are some tips for closing the group.

- After the relaxation segment, look around the group and acknowledge the efforts of each participant.
- Thank everyone for coming and participating.
- This is a good time to review safety and educational tips. Ask the participants if they have any questions or areas needing further review.
- Be sure to address progress and accomplishments. Feedback is very important.

- Remind participants of the next session date and time. Remind participants about any specific exercises that you recommend they do before the next session.
- After you close the group officially, begin to assist individual participants. Some participants may need you to get their walkers, which may have been placed behind the chairs or to the side of the room. Always check the name to be sure that participants are walking away with the correct walkers, canes, and personal belongings.
- Complete the attendance board chart while the group is still together.
- Be sure that you have collected all supplies, weights, water bottles, and towels.
- Look around to ensure that no one has forgotten any personal adaptive devices or equipment.
- If you are playing music, keep it on low until all participants have left.
- You want each resident to leave feeling positive about the experience, themselves, and you. The success that they feel will motivate them to return. As a fitness leader, you can help participants feel successful by giving positive and clear feedback.

FEEDBACK

One of your most important roles as the fitness leader is to give feedback to your participants. The frail elderly and those with special needs are often unaware of their progress, especially if they are insecure about or lack confidence in their physical abilities. They need someone else's verbal reinforcement to help them see how well they are doing.

Feedback can be both general and individual. General feedback is for the entire class; for example, "In the past two months, each of you has gained flexibility. We can see this when we compare your arm flexibility with the initial pretest." Individual feedback pertains to one participant; for example, "Ms. Jones, I wanted to comment on how much improvement I see in your ability to complete the balance exercises without holding onto the chair." The feedback that you give needs to be specific and concrete. It should be given when you observe a change or improvement. By doing so, you can correct improper form before it becomes a habit. Individual feedback can also be given one-on-one after class. This is a good idea for participants who are easily embarrassed in the group setting.

Some of your participants' progress may seem slow and, at times, unlikely. If a participant feels discouraged, he or she should look first at the length of his or her involvement in the class. You can count on the board how many sessions he or she has attended and mention the progress reflected on the board. This takes your feedback from general to the specific individual's own progress. Our class has gone through a few attendance boards (see figure 3.3). Just having a new board is a positive statement for the individual participants along with the groups as a whole. These boards reflect changes in fitness also. Sometimes just reviewing and reminding participants about their improvements helps them see that they are meeting fitness goals. Even newer participants feel encouraged with the results that they see with other members. Keep your old attendance records to track long-term progress.

Another way of providing feedback and tracking progress is to take photographs at different times.

One of our participants, Anita, had a right-side cerebrovascular accident (stroke) that affected her entire left side. When Anita started the exercise class, she had no movement in her left arm. We encouraged her to keep a soft ball in her left hand and try to squeeze it. She also would move her left arm with her right hand during exercises. After six months, she was feeling discouraged and saw no improvement. We were able to show her before and after photos that told the story better than any words could have. Her left arm was moving through almost 90 percent range of motion, compared with an initial no range of motion.

All feedback needs to be honest and genuine. Be aware that some individuals do not take recommendations well. Always focus on the positive and acknowledge improvement. Then mention any recommendations, and finish with a compliment. This balances progress made in the past with the goals to work toward in the future.

FINISHING TOUCHES: ORGANIZING SUPPLIES AND TAKING ATTENDANCE

Your class is over for the day. After helping participants gather their things and saying good-bye, you are now ready for the finishing touches: reorganizing the supplies and taking attendance for the day. It is most ideal to take attendance while participants are present. But, some of you may complete more detailed attendance logs after the official ending of the class or after organizing the supplies and equipment. Attendance records should include dates, attendance, and exercise details, such as length of aerobic component, sets, repetitions, and weights used (see appendix K).

You have many things to remember that you want to jot down. But first, take care of the physical environment and supplies. On the next page is a checklist of things to do after class.

SUMMARY

This chapter is for and about you, the fitness leader. Success as a fitness leader begins with creating a sense of fun and community within your group. Participants join an exercise class for a variety of reasons. Some come to exercise, while others are looking for new friends. You, as the leader, create an environment that can nurture friendships and social support. Never forget the importance of fun. Fun brings back the enjoyment of new experiences and the rapture of being human.

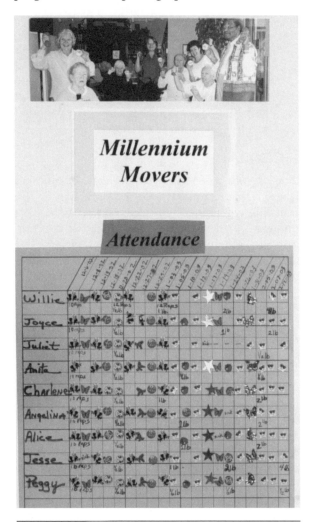

FIGURE 3.3   Attendance records and boards.

Finishing Touches Checklist

❑ Once the participants have departed, organize the supplies and equipment. You should have an inventory sheet that itemizes everything you brought to class. Ensure that each item is accounted for.

❑ Supplies and weights used in the class should be sprayed down with a mixture of equal parts water and alcohol. Place them on a towel and leave them to dry while you organize the other supplies. All supplies should be clean, properly stored, and ready for the next class.

❑ Depending on the setting of your exercise class, there may be little time between activity groups. Be sure to give your participants ample time to depart and yourself ample time to get organized before the next event.

From *Exercise for Frail Elders* by E. Best-Martini and K. A. Botenhagen-DiGenova, 2003, Champaign, IL: Human Kinetics.

Another important responsibility is setting up the group exercise class, from setting up the room, organizing the supplies and equipment, to deciding whether to use music or not. This may seem simplistic to the new leader, but the experienced leader knows that good organization is the basis for a successful class experience. Your participants will feel more secure and confident in you when they can see that you are well prepared.

Next we discussed helpful tips for opening your class. We all know that first impressions are important. Many of your participants will feel nervous or a little anxious about starting to exercise. You need to make them feel welcome and to begin building their confidence. Your participants look to you as a role model and for guidance, support, and consistency. Your safety and educational reminders during the class reinforce the exercise and its relationship to functional skills needed in their everyday lives.

Successfully leading the exercise class starts with a safe and effective instructional routine. The three-step instructional process works hand in hand with specific techniques for teaching participants with communication, cognitive, and sensory losses. These techniques have been successful in our work with frail elderly participants and adults with special needs for many years.

Finally, we presented helpful tips for closing your exercise class. You can use this time to give feedback both to the group and to individual participants. The "Finishing Touches Checklist" provides tips for organizing after your class and preparing for the next class.

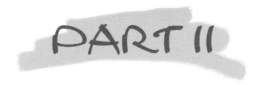

PART II

IMPLEMENTING AN EXERCISE PROGRAM FOR FRAIL ELDERS AND ADULTS WITH SPECIAL NEEDS

In chapters 4 through 7, you will find warm-up, aerobic, resistance, and cool-down exercises, respectively. Along with the exercises are simple teaching instructions to get you started and variations and progression options to keep your exercise classes interesting for repeat participants. Each exercise has a seated position and a standing variation. Many frail elders and adults with special needs are able to stand but not get up off the floor; therefore, floor exercises are not included. In chapter 8, you will learn how to put warm-up, aerobic, resistance, and cool-down exercises together into a safe and effective fitness program. A primary goal of this exercise program is to promote *functional fitness* (a person's ability to perform daily activities). Although we geared this part of the book toward class or group instruction, the information presented is also useful when working one-on-one with this population.

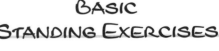

Chapters 4 through 7 cover the following topics:

- Safety precautions
- Exercise guidelines
- Basic seated exercises
- Basic standing exercises
- Variations and progression
- An illustrated instructional guide to exercises

Chapter 8 is packed with ideas for creating fun, varied, and progressive exercise routines for your participants.

BASIC SEATED EXERCISES

The basic seated exercises are ideal for individuals just beginning an exercise program, particularly those in wheelchairs or who are at risk of falling when they stand. The exercises can be performed in wheelchairs or chairs with or without arms. However, chairs without arms are preferable if they are safe for a participant, because they allow greater range of motion of the limbs. These exercises are also ideal for instructors—beginning and experienced—who are getting to know their participants' strengths and limitations. Seated exercises eliminate concerns over participants' falling. As participants improve their muscular strength and endurance with the seated exercises, they also improve their ability and stamina for standing exercises.

BASIC STANDING EXERCISES

Each basic seated exercise has a standing alternative. We discuss in chapter 8 the benefits of the standing variations and when the seated versions are preferred. Even participants who can do the standing exercises have the option of doing them seated instead, especially if they are feeling fatigued or unsteady on their feet. You may choose to lead some exercises, such as the warm-up, in the seated position and then lead the rest in the standing position. If one or more participants are unable to exercise standing, it is easier to initiate an exercise class with everyone seated and then progress at a comfortable pace. When a participant is ready to do standing exercises, he or she can start with one or two standing exercises and gradually progress to as many as are comfortable. Participants can sit down and rejoin the others who are doing the seated exercises if they become fatigued and stand again when they are ready. The basic seated and standing exercises are designed to be taught at the same time, so your exercise class can accommodate various needs.

VARIATIONS AND PROGRESSION

We provide variations and progression options for each basic seated range-of-motion, aerobic, resistance, and stretching exercise. You may introduce these exercises after your participants have learned the basic seated exercises. Some classes—for example, a large class without an assistant in a long-term care facility—may offer limited opportunity for extensive *progression* (progressively more challenging exercise), but varying the basic seated exercises can add pizzazz to your class. Other classes may outgrow the seated exercises and be able to do a standing workout. Standing exercises offer participants the greatest benefits for functional mobility and increased independence. Chapters 4 through 7 show variations and progression options for each exercise component. You will find many other ideas for varying and progressing the exercises in chapter 8, which includes sections on designing, scheduling, progressing, and maintaining a smart fitness program. The variations and progression options enable you to be creative and flexible with your fitness program over the years and to tailor your program to meet participants' needs.

ILLUSTRATED INSTRUCTION GUIDE

The instruction guides at the end of chapters 4 through 7 have a consistent format for illustrating and describing each basic seated exercise:

- A concise description and photograph(s) of the exercise
- Exercise and safety tips
- Variations and progression options

A photograph and description is provided for standing exercises and other variations and progression options that need further explanation.

PUTTING THE EXERCISES TOGETHER

Chapter 8 gives practical information for leading an exercise class, such as

- how to extend a single warm-up, aerobic, resistance-training, or stretching component into an entire class;
- how to design your class for a variety of fitness levels and special needs;
- determining when a participant is ready for standing exercises;
- when seated exercises are preferred over standing ones;
- how to teach the seated and standing exercise at the same time;
- when to introduce intermediate-level ("challenger") exercises or the variations and progressions; and
- how to integrate warm-up, aerobic, resistance, and cool-down exercises into a comprehensive fitness program.

With the exception of the aerobic exercises, we recommend that all exercises be done in the order given. However, you may instead alternate upper- and lower-body exercises, which helps to prevent fatigue and adds variety to your fitness class. You can do one or more upper-body exercises and then alternate with one or more lower-body exercises. Find a pattern that is easy to remember. The exercises are numbered to help you keep track of where you are.

This part will help you to confidently and competently teach seated and standing warm-up, aerobic, resistance, and cool-down exercises. You will also learn how to put together a dynamic fitness program and to vary and progress your classes so that they are fun and functional.

CHAPTER 4

WARM-UP FIRST: POSTURE, BREATHING, RANGE-OF-MOTION, AND STRETCHING EXERCISES

This chapter provides practical safety precautions, guidelines, and teaching instructions for the warm-up period before exercise. The warm-up exercises focus on joint range-of-motion (ROM) exercises and include posture, breathing, and stretching exercises. Always have your participants warm up to prepare them for exercise and to help prevent muscle and joint injury. Start with the basic seated warm-up exercises, which all your participants can learn. Participants who are able to stand safely can carefully progress to the basic standing warm-up exercises. The seated and standing exercises are designed to be taught at the same time. Figure 4.1 illustrates how manageable it is to lead the seated and standing exercises simultaneously. Photographs and descriptions of the warm-up ROM exercises are at the end of this chapter.

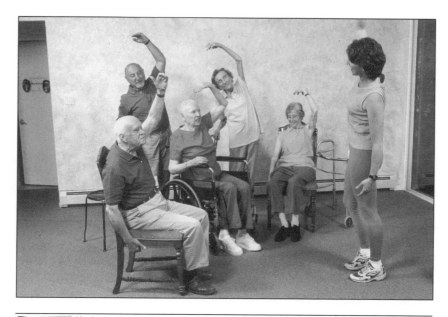

FIGURE 4.1 Seated and standing exercises can be taught at the same time.

SAFETY PRECAUTIONS FOR WARM-UPS

Warm-up exercises are safe for older adults when appropriate guidelines and precautions are observed. The following general safety precautions and specific safety precautions for those with special needs can help you lead safe warm-ups and keep your participants injury-free. You may photocopy the following "General Safety Precautions Checklist for Warm-Ups" and the general exercise "Safety Guidelines Checklist" in chapter 2.

SPECIFIC SAFETY PRECAUTIONS FOR THOSE WITH SPECIAL NEEDS

Your class can focus on one or more special needs. For example, you might lead a class for individuals with arthritis, multiple sclerosis, or any condition likely to decrease normal *range of motion* (the degree of movement that occurs at a joint). Such a group could greatly benefit from a mild ROM program that gently moves every joint through its full, pain-free range of motion daily. Teaching participants with similar special needs as opposed to a class with a variety of special needs can be an easier way to start a class, though not always possible.

Following are some safety precautions for leading warm-up exercises for people with specific needs. They may not apply to every individual with a particular medical condition. For example, an individual with mild symptoms of multiple sclerosis may have no limitations on ROM exercises, whereas severe symptoms may cause difficulty with all ROM exercises. Also, remember that an individual's performance ability can vary from day to day. See chapter 1 to learn more about common medical disorders in the elderly. Above all, follow the physician's or physical therapist's special exercise recommendations for the participant.

General Safety Precautions Checklist for Warm-Ups

❑ Review the physician's or physical therapist's comments and special recommendations for each participant on the "Statement of Medical Clearance for Exercise" (appendix C).

❑ Remind participants to observe recommendations from their physicians or physical therapists.

❑ Never skip the warm-up period. If a participant is late for class and misses the warm-up, he or she should do whatever activity the class is doing at a lower intensity for 10 minutes. For example, the participant can do resistance exercises without weights or aerobics at a low intensity for 10 minutes.

❑ Always spend at least 10 minutes on warm-up exercises.

❑ The back should be warmed up in a vertical position before twisting or bending the trunk sideways.

❑ During upper- and lower-body ROM exercises, participants should lift arms and legs only as high as comfortable while maintaining erect posture.

❑ Participants should avoid *hyperextending* (locking or extending a limb or part beyond the normal joint ROM). When standing, they should avoid locking the knee of the supporting leg; they should keep the knee soft, not bent.

❑ Continually encourage your participants to maintain good posture and breathing (no breath holding) while exercising.

❑ Focus on fun and safety!

ARTHRITIS

- A thorough warm-up is especially important for participants with arthritis. Their joints need extra time to reduce stiffness and prepare for exercise that is more vigorous.
- To maintain joint ROM and mobility, those with arthritis should perform warm-up and stretching exercises daily (one to two sessions per day), even when *inflammation* (redness, heat, swelling and pain) is present.
- When a joint is significantly inflamed, the participant should perform only one or two slow and gentle ROM exercises, moving through a comfortable or functional ROM. For instance, although 90 degrees is a normal wrist flexion range, a range of only about 45 degrees is needed for daily activities.
- If mild ROM exercises exacerbate inflamed joints, rest may be needed.

CEREBROVASCULAR ACCIDENT (STROKE)

- Perform three to five repetitions of each ROM exercise.

CHRONIC OBSTRUCTIVE PULMONARY DISEASE (COPD)

- A thorough warm-up period is critical for participants with COPD. Their respiratory and cardiovascular systems need extra time to adapt to changes in physical exertion.
- Arm ROM exercises can cause shortness of breath sooner than leg ROM exercises. If you combine arm and leg exercises, give participants permission to do just the leg exercises; this results in a better warm-up than arm exercises alone.

- Remind participants with COPD to practice *diaphragmatic breathing* (see "Instructions for First-Stage Breathing" later in this chapter) with *pursed-lip breathing* (see the following "Instructions for Pursed-Lip Breathing") while exercising. If a participant is experiencing *dyspnea* (difficulty breathing, with rapid shallow respirations) or *hyperventilation* (increased rate and depth of breathing), have him or her stop exercise and just practice the breathing.

CORONARY ARTERY DISEASE (HEART DISEASE)

- A thorough warm-up is critical for participants with cardiovascular problems that limit the heart's oxygen supply. The warm-up serves two purposes: (1) It reduces *myocardial* (heart muscle) workload and thus oxygen requirement, and (2) it enhances blood flow to the heart.

HIP FRACTURE OR REPLACEMENT

- When the participant receives medical clearance for a maintenance exercise program, you should strive to maintain the degree of muscle control and ROM that the participant achieved in physical therapy and progress from there.
- Avoid ROM exercises that involve *internal rotation* (turning the leg inward), *hip adduction* (crossing the legs), and hip flexion of more than 90 degrees (thigh higher than parallel with the floor) to reduce the risk of hip dislocation. If a participant is sitting in a chair that allows the knees to be lower than the hips and the participant is able to follow instructions, he or she may raise the foot 1 inch (2.5 centimeters) off the floor during the following exercises: Seated Up-and-Down Leg March, Seated

---

INSTRUCTIONS FOR PURSED-LIP BREATHING[a]

1. Breathe in slowly through your nose. Keep your mouth closed.
2. Pucker (purse) your lips as if you were going to whistle.
3. Breathe out slowly through your pursed lips.[b]
4. Repeat several times or until breathing calms.

Encourage participants with COPD to practice this technique throughout the day.

[a]Participants should first practice pursed-lip breathing alone and then combine it with diaphragmatic breathing (see "Instructions for First-Stage Breathing" later in this chapter).

[b]The exhalation should take two to three times as long as the inhalation. Start with a 2-second inhalation and a 4-second exhalation.

Out-and-In Leg March, and Seated Hip Rotation. During the Seated Out-and-In Leg March, a participant can slide the foot out and in rather than lift the leg. Also, instruct the participant to do only small circles (avoid leaning forward) during the Seated and the Standing Torso Rotation.

Multiple Sclerosis and Parkinson's Disease

- Range of motion can be significantly reduced for those with these chronic neurologic conditions. Encourage participants to do the version of each ROM exercise that best serves them.

- Anyone with any trouble controlling neck movement should avoid neck ROM exercises because of the increased risk of injury.

- When performing upper-body ROM exercises and combined upper- and lower-body ROM exercises, the participant should be seated in a chair.

Osteoporosis

- Avoid ROM exercises that involve *spinal flexion* (bending forward at the waist), particularly in combination with stooping, which increases the risk of vertebral fractures (ACSM 1997, 163). Have the participant do only the "Mellow Cat" (gentle backward arch) portion, not the "Mad Cat" (spinal flexion), of Mad and Mellow Cat, and do only small circles (avoid leaning forward) with Torso Rotation.

Sensory Losses

- Give a clear demonstration of the warm-up exercises to participants with hearing loss.

- Describe warm-up exercises precisely and directly to participants with visual impairment.

Guidelines for Warm-Ups

Begin every workout with a warm-up. A 10-minute warm-up is essential for increasing blood flow to the exercising muscles, raising deep muscle temperature, loosening up muscles and joints, increasing joint ROM and function, and helping prevent muscle and joint injury. Table 4.1 shows the duration of various parts of a 10- to 15-minute warm-up. The warm-up exercises are shown in the recommended order, beginning with posture awareness,

TABLE 4.1 Duration of the Segments of a 10- to 15-Minute Warm-Up	
Warm-up exercises	**Duration**
1. Posture awareness	1/2 to 1 minute
2. Two-part deep breathing	1/2 to 1 minute
3. Joint range of motion[a]	8 to 10 minutes
4. Stretching	1 to 3 minutes

[a]Low-intensity aerobic exercises (see chapter 5) may replace or be combined with joint ROM exercises.

then two-part deep-breathing, joint ROM, and finally stretching.

Please note that, even if your class starts late, you should still do at least a 10-minute warm-up. Also, if you plan to lead both resistance and aerobic exercises in a class, the group needs to warm up only in the beginning if aerobics precede resistance training. If you lead resistance exercises before aerobics, stretch briefly (using the minimal five stretching exercises in table 4.3; see page 66) immediately after resistance training and follow with several minutes of active rhythmic movement (such as slow walking or low-intensity aerobic leg exercises) before moving on to the aerobic workout.

A well-rounded initial warm-up for frail elders and adults with special needs includes posture, deep-breathing, joint ROM, and stretching exercises. The following guidelines for each segment apply to leading both seated and standing exercises.

Posture-Awareness Guidelines

Good posture is crucial. Poor posture reduces range of motion and breathing capacity and increases the risk of falling and incidence of pain, particularly in the low back. You can inspire participants' enthusiasm for exercise by taking them from a slumped to an upright posture.

Keep the following guidelines in mind when leading the posture-awareness exercise:

- Teach the posture-awareness exercise first, so your participants can begin exercise with improved posture. (See the sections "Seated Posture-Awareness Exercise" and "Standing Posture-Awareness Exercise" later in this chapter.)

- In the initial stages of teaching the exercises, give a quick reminder about good posture between warm-up, aerobic, resistance, and cool-down exercises.

- When participants have learned the exercises and you flow from exercise to exercise without pausing, give a posture lesson at the beginning of class and reminders when needed.

- When you observe a participant slumping or overarching the back, try these tips:

  1. Give a general reminder about good posture to the class.

  2. Use positive terms, such as "lift" or "open your chest," as opposed to "don't slump."

  3. Give specific encouragement to the participant if he or she still needs it after the general reminder.

- Never physically force anybody into good posture.

- Instruct participants to not hold the body in a rigid or static posture. Promote a relaxed and lifted posture by having participants gently shake their arms after the posture exercise.

- If a participant tends to lift the shoulders while doing the ROM exercises, have him or her stabilize the shoulders by moving them up, back, and down to help keep the shoulders down throughout each exercise.

- Visual imagery can be helpful. For example, to convey the idea of the spine getting longer when sitting or standing erect, say, "Imagine your spine as a piece of elastic thread being pulled out from the top of your head at the same time that it is being pulled at its base" (Diamond 1996, 4).

- Look for opportunities to tell the group, "Your posture is looking good."

- Give individuals positive feedback when working one-on-one or before or after class.

- Encourage your participants to sit erect using postural muscles and not to rest their backs against the backs of their chairs for as long as possible throughout the exercise class. Instruct them to scoot their buttocks to the back of the chair when they get tired and need support (to minimize slumping).

Two-Part Deep-Breathing Guidelines

The two-part deep-breathing exercise (see the section "Seated Two-Part Deep-Breathing Exercise" later in this chapter) improves mental focus, which can help your participants concentrate better on your instructions and thus avoid injury. Here are a few simple guidelines for leading the two-part deep-breathing exercise:

- Do deep breathing before exercise to relax participants and make them more aware of their bodies.

- Instruct participants never to hold their breath.

- If a participant feels light-headed or dizzy during the two-part deep-breathing, he or she should resume a normal breathing rhythm. If the participant is standing, he or she should sit down.

- Try to integrate deep breathing into the exercise session, for example, one two-part deep breath between each resistance exercise.

- Throughout the class, remind participants to sit with good posture and to keep breathing.

Joint Range-of-Motion Guidelines

Continuous, rhythmic ROM exercises are excellent for gently preparing frail elders and individuals with special needs for exercise. See the sections "Seated Joint Range-of-Motion Exercises," "Standing Joint Range-of-Motion Exercises," and "Illustrated Range-of-Motion Instruction" later in this chapter. ROM exercises also help improve flexibility, musculoskeletal function, balance, and agility in older adults. The joint ROM exercises work all the major joints of the body. Follow these guidelines when leading ROM exercises:

- Begin with six to eight *repetitions* (the number of times an exercise is performed without a break) of each ROM exercise, if well tolerated by participants. Starting with fewer repetitions may not give you enough time to observe and evaluate all participants and give them appropriate feedback about each exercise (see "Three-Step Instructional Process" in chapter 3).

- After the exercises are familiar to the participants, you may lower the number of repetitions to three or four if you need extra time for aerobics, resistance training, or stretching.

- Do not rest between ROM exercises. Keep the movement continuous to increase the internal body temperature, which is a primary goal of warm-ups.

- Gradually increase the speed and *intensity* (how hard you're exercising) of the warm-up exercises during a class. To increase the intensity of warm-up exercises, make larger movements, but keep the movements within all individuals' pain-free ROM.

- As always, encourage participants to stop when they are fatigued. When a participant is tired, remind him or her, "Stop, rest, and rejoin us when you are ready."

- Each repetition is about 1 second in each direction of the ROM exercise, compared with 3 seconds for resistance exercises.

- Perform warm-up ROM exercises slowly and smoothly.

- Do not use dumbbells or other resistance props with ROM exercises.

- Initially, it can be easier for participants to learn a ROM exercise by doing six to eight repetitions on one side at a time. This way participants can properly learn an exercise on one side at a time, before coordinating both sides simultaneously. There are two exceptions:

  1. Hip exercises (marching in place)
  2. Wrist exercises and toe and heel raises: Do both sides together.

- After your participants are comfortable with the ROM exercises on one side, you can use one of these movement patterns:

  1. Alternate sides.
  2. Exercise both arms together.

Safety Tip

Do not exercise both legs at one time. One foot should always be planted firmly on the floor while exercising the other leg to help prevent lower-back strain.

  3. Ultimately, for a more effective warm-up, do upper- and lower-body ROM exercises together (e.g., leg march plus butterfly wings). See chapter 5 for upper- and lower-body aerobic exercises that can be performed at a low intensity as a warm-up.

- For a more effective warm-up, include more exercises that use larger muscles, such as marching, between upper-body exercises. To keep the warm-up a reasonable length, do only three to five repetitions of each exercise.

Safety Tip

Avoid doing too many ROM exercises that focus on small muscle groups, such as wrist and finger

exercises, which can delay the goal of warming up the body.

- You may replace the ROM segment of the warm-up with low-impact, low-intensity aerobic activity, such as walking or stationary cycling. Incorporate some upper-body ROM exercises while walking or cycling, as long as participants can do them safely.

- Add some spice to the warm-ups with the variations and progression options in the "Illustrated Range-of-Motion Instruction" section.

STRETCHING GUIDELINES

Warm-up, or preactivity, stretching is intended to prepare the body for exercise, whereas cool-down, or postactivity, stretching promotes flexibility. (See the sections "Seated Stretching Exercises" and "Standing Stretching Exercises" later in this chapter.) Here are guidelines for leading the warm-up stretches (for more details on stretching, see chapter 7):

- Do stretching at the end of the warm-up, after posture, breathing, and ROM exercises.

- Remember to stretch only warmed-up muscles to avoid injuring cold muscles and joints.

- During the warm-up, do a shorter set of stretching exercises (table 4.3 or 4.4) than during the cool-down. Tables 4.3 and 4.4 include critical stretches for body parts that are notoriously tight for the majority of older adults. Tightness can compromise posture, impair balance, and reduce functional mobility.

- Hold warm-up stretches for 10 seconds. (During the cool-down, do more stretches, and hold them for 15 to 30 seconds.)

BASIC SEATED WARM-UP EXERCISES

The basic seated warm-up focuses on joint ROM exercises but also includes posture, breathing, and stretching exercises. Before teaching these exercises, be sure to review the guidelines and safety precautions for warm-up exercises. Also, if you are a beginner fitness leader or would like to refine your leadership skills, review the three-step instructional process in chapter 3. Begin teaching the basic seated warm-up exercises before the basic standing warm-up exercises. Participants who are able to stand safely can slowly progress to the standing versions.

SEATED POSTURE-AWARENESS EXERCISE

Teach good seated posture first to get participants in the habit of exercising with good posture (see "Instructions for Good Seated Posture" below). A primary objective of the posture exercise is to find the natural curves of the spine—a *neutral spine* (figure 4.2). You may enlarge figure 4.2 to use as a visual aid for your class. You know you have achieved a neutral spine when you are sitting as tall as possible with a long and lifted spine. Remind participants to maintain this improved posture throughout the class and throughout the day. Verbally explain and physically demonstrate good seated posture. You may also copy the instructions for reference during class.

If a participant's feet cannot reach the floor, have him or her scoot forward in the chair. If he or she is unable to sustain that position, provide a foot support, such as a sturdy box lid, a phone book, or a folded towel.

SEATED TWO-PART DEEP-BREATHING EXERCISE

Teach two-part deep-breathing in two stages. Start with first-stage breathing. After your participants are comfortable with first-stage breathing (this may take one class or several weeks), add second-stage breathing. If your warm-up is the minimum 10 minutes, lead a short posture and breathing segment of about 1 minute. In this case, you do only about three deep breaths. The posture and breathing exercises come before the ROM exercises. Whether you start with lower- or upper-body ROM exercises, do posture and breathing exercises first.

Step-by-step instructions for teaching two-part deep-breathing are shown in the boxes on p. 64. The instructions apply in both the seated and standing

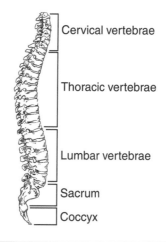

Cervical vertebrae

Thoracic vertebrae

Lumbar vertebrae

Sacrum

Coccyx

FIGURE 4.2 The natural curves of the spine.

Reprinted, by permission, from E. Aabert, 1998, *Muscle mechanics* (Champaign, IL: Human Kinetics), 36.

INSTRUCTIONS FOR GOOD SEATED POSTURE

1. Hips: Move your hips to the back of your chair. Sit with your spine erect. Do not lean against the back of the chair.[a]

2. Feet: Place your feet on the floor about hip distance apart, toes pointed forward. Take care that both the heels and balls of your feet are touching the floor.

3. Knees: Adjust your foot placement so that your knees are directly over your ankles.

4. Hands: Place your hands on your thighs.

5. Chest: Take a big breath, and feel your chest lift and expand. Maintain that lifted feeling.

6. Shoulders: Shrug, and then relax your shoulders while maintaining erect posture (see Seated Shoulder Shrugs, exercise 4.17). Repeat as needed.

7. Head and neck: Keep the bottom of your chin parallel with the floor.

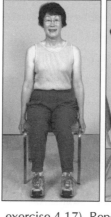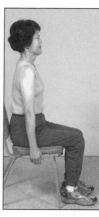

Check each participant for good seated posture.

Visualization: To help maintain good posture, imagine a string attached to the top of your head, pulling gently. Your torso is lengthening with ease.

[a]Leaning against the back of a chair usually results in slumping and flattening of the lower-back curve. To help maintain good seated posture, place a rolled hand towel (wrapped with rubber bands) behind the lower back. The roll should be about 3 inches (8 centimeters) thick (depending on body size) to support the natural curve of the lower back.

From *Exercise for Frail Elders* by E. Best-Martini and K. A. Botenhagen-DiGenova, 2003, Champaign, IL: Human Kinetics.

INSTRUCTIONS FOR FIRST-STAGE BREATHING

1. Exhale fully.

2. Inhale and allow the abdomen to expand like a balloon filling up with air. (You may want to place your hand on your abdomen and feel the muscles move out.)

3. Exhale and pull the abdomen in toward the spine. (Feel the abdominal muscles tighten, squeezing out more air from the lungs.)

First-Stage Breathing

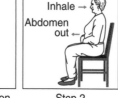

Beginning position   Step 2   Step 3

4. Continue for about five or six breaths at a rhythm you find comfortable. (Be sure the abdomen goes out on the inhalation, in on the exhalation.)

5. On the final exhalation, relax. You have completed the first stage of this breathing practice.

Adapted, by permission, from M.D. Scheller, 1993, *Growing older, feeling better in body, mind and spirit* (Palo Alto, CA: Bull), 19. From *Exercise for Frail Elders* by E. Best-Martini and K. A. Botenhagen-DiGenova, 2003, Champaign, IL: Human Kinetics.

INSTRUCTIONS FOR SECOND-STAGE BREATHING

1. To begin second-stage breathing, exhale fully.

2. Inhale and feel your abdomen expand, as in first-stage breathing.

3. Keep inhaling and feel your rib cage expand. (You may want to place your hand on your rib cage.)

4. When you exhale, feel the rib cage contract.

5. Now pull in the abdomen toward the spine.

6. Continue for about five or six breaths at your own rate and rhythm. You are doing two-part breathing.

Second-Stage Breathing

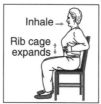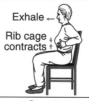

Step 8   Step 9

7. On the last exhalation, relax. You have completed the second stage of this breathing practice.

Adapted, by permission, from M.D. Scheller, 1993, *Growing older, feeling better in body, mind and spirit* (Palo Alto, CA: Bull), 20. From *Exercise for Frail Elders* by E. Best-Martini and K. A. Botenhagen-DiGenova, 2003, Champaign, IL: Human Kinetics.

positions. Verbally explain and physically demonstrate first-stage breathing and second-stage breathing. You may copy these two sets of instructions to refer to during class.

SEATED JOINT RANGE-OF-MOTION EXERCISES

The 24 seated joint ROM exercises are carefully organized to help you and your participants remember these exercises. You may make a copy of table 4.2 to refer to during class, which lists the exercises in a preferred order. However, warm up the back by performing 4.18 Rowing and 4.19 Close the Window before the spine ROM exercises, until participants learn 4.7 Mad and Mellow Cat (challenger).

This is the general order of ROM exercises for each joint:

1. Up and down or forward and backward movement: flexion and extension (*Extension* is movement that increases the joint angle between adjacent body parts. *Flexion* is movement that decreases the joint angle between adjacent body parts.)

2. Sideward movement: abduction and adduction (*Abduction* is sideward movement away from the body. *Adduction* is sideward movement towards the body.)

3. Circular movement: rotation

4. Additional movements possible for a specific joint

Additionally, the ROM exercises systematically cover the entire upper and lower body. You may start with either the lower- or the upper-body ROM exercises.

TABLE 4.2	BASIC SEATED WARM-UP[a]	
		Page
Posture exercise	See "Instructions for Good Seated Posture" in this chapter	63
Breathing exercise	See "Instructions for First-Stage Breathing" and "Instructions for Second-Stage Breathing" in this chapter	64, 64
Target joints	**Seated Lower-Body Range-of-Motion Exercises**	
Hips	4.1 Seated Up-and-Down Leg March	69
	4.2 Seated Out-and-In Leg March	70
	4.3 Seated Hip Rotation	71
Knees	4.4 Seated Best Foot Forward and Backward	72
Ankles	4.5 Seated Toe Point and Flex	73
	4.6 Seated Ankle Rotations	74
Target joints	**Seated Upper-Body Range-of-Motion Exercises**	
Spine	4.7 Seated Mad and Mellow Cat (challenger)	75
	4.8 Seated Side Reach	76
	4.9 Seated Torso Rotation	77
	4.10 Seated Twists	78
Cervical spine (neck)	4.11 Seated Chin to Chest ("Yes")	79
	4.12 Seated Chin to Shoulder	80
Shoulders	4.13 Seated Arm Swing	81
	4.14 Seated Butterfly Wings	82
	4.15 Seated Shoulder Rotation	83
	4.16 Seated Stir the Soup	84
	4.17 Seated Shoulder Shrugs	85
Shoulders and elbows	4.18 Seated Rowing	86
	4.19 Seated Close the Window	87
Wrists	4.20 Seated Wrist Flexion and Extension	88
	4.21 Seated Wrist Rotations	89
Fingers	4.22 Seated Hands Open and Closed	90
	4.23 Seated Sun Rays	91
	4.24 Seated Piano Playing	92
Seated Warm-Up Stretches		
"The Minimal Five Stretching Exercises" (table 4.3) or "Eight Warm-Up Stretches" (table 4.4)		66, 66

[a]Seated upper- and lower-body warm-ups can be adapted to standing exercises.
From *Exercise for Frail Elders* by E. Best-Martini and K. A. Botenhagen-DiGenova, 2003, Champaign, IL: Human Kinetics.

Before leading the seated ROM exercises, note the following tips:

- Review the general exercise "Safety Guidelines Checklist" (in chapter 2) and the section "Safety Precautions for Warm-Ups" (earlier in this chapter) before leading these exercises.

- Review the photographs, teaching instructions, and variations and progression options at the end of this chapter.

- Seated upper- and lower-body warm-ups can be adapted to standing exercises. See the section "Standing Joint Range-of-Motion Exercises" later in this chapter.

- You can do either the lower- or upper-body ROM exercises first; do a posture and breathing exercise before the ROM exercises.

- Do the challenger (intermediate-level exercise), Seated Mad and Mellow Cat, after participants are comfortable with the other basic seated exercises.

SEATED STRETCHING EXERCISES

Teach seated stretching exercises after the ROM exercises, when your participants are warmed up. Two sets of warm-up stretching exercises for you to choose from appear in table 4.3, "The Minimal Five Stretching Exercises," and table 4.4, "Eight Warm-Up Stretches," both of which are shorter than the comprehensive set of 12 stretching exercises in chapter 7. All the stretching exercises are illustrated and described in chapter 7, which also gives safety tips and variations and progression options for each stretch. You may copy tables 4.3 and 4.4 for use during class.

TABLE 4.3 The Minimal Five Stretching Exercises

Basic Seated Stretching Exercises[a]	Page	Basic Standing Stretching Exercises[b]	Page
7.3 Seated Swan	163	7.3 Standing Swan	163
7.8 Seated Tib Touches	168	7.8 Standing Tib Touches	169
7.5 Seated Zipper Stretch	165	7.5 Standing Zipper Stretch	165
7.12 Seated Calf Stretch	174	7.12 Standing Calf Stretch	175
7.7 Seated Spinal Twist	167	7.7 Standing Spinal Twist	167

Stretches are in a recommended but optional order, alternating upper- and lower-body stretches.

[a]Refer to table 7.3 and the "Illustrated Stretching Instruction" in chapter 7.

[b]Refer to table 7.4 and the "Illustrated Stretching Instruction" in chapter 7.

From *Exercise for Frail Elders* by E. Best-Martini and K. A. Botenhagen-DiGenova, 2003, Champaign, IL: Human Kinetics.

TABLE 4.4 Eight Warm-Up Stretches

Basic Seated Stretching Exercises[a]	Page	Basic Standing Stretching Exercises[b]	Page
7.3 Seated Swan	163	7.3 Standing Swan	163
7.5 Seated Zipper Stretch	165	7.5 Standing Zipper Stretch	165
7.7 Seated Spinal Twist	167	7.7 Standing Spinal Twist	167
7.8 Seated Tib Touches	168	7.8 Standing Tib Touches	169
7.9 Seated Quad Stretch	169	7.9 Standing Quad Stretch (challenger)[c]	170
7.10 Seated Splits	171	7.10 Standing Half-Splits	172
7.11 Seated Outer-Thigh Stretch	172	7.11 Standing Outer-Thigh Stretch	173
7.12 Seated Calf Stretch	174	7.12 Standing Calf Stretch	175

[a]Refer to table 7.3 and the "Illustrated Stretching Instruction" in chapter 7.

[b]Refer to table 7.4 and the "Illustrated Stretching Instruction" in chapter 7.

[c]If a participant has trouble with the Standing Quad Stretch, or any of the standing exercises, he or she can do the corresponding seated stretch.

From *Exercise for Frail Elders* by E. Best-Martini and K. A. Botenhagen-DiGenova, 2003, Champaign, IL: Human Kinetics.

BASIC STANDING WARM-UP EXERCISES

The basic standing warm-up, like the seated one, focuses on ROM exercises and includes posture, breathing, and stretching exercises. These exercises can replace the basic seated warm-ups, or both can be taught at the same time. We recommend that anyone who cannot safely stand continue with the seated warm-up exercises. Participants with *minor* balance problems should perform only those standing exercises that leave one hand available to hold on to the back of the chair for support. ROM exercises that use two hands should be performed only by participants who are steady on their feet. Here are instructions for leading the basic standing warm-ups in the recommended order: first posture, then breathing, ROM exercises, and finally stretching after the body is warmed up.

STANDING POSTURE-AWARENESS EXERCISE

Teach good standing posture (see instructions in the box below) to those who are doing standing exercises to get them in the habit of exercising with good posture. A primary objective of the posture exercise is to find the natural curves of the spine, when you are standing as tall as possible (see figure 4.2). Remind participants to maintain this improved posture throughout the class and throughout the day. Explain and physically demonstrate good standing posture. You may copy the instructions to refer to during class.

STANDING TWO-PART DEEP-BREATHING EXERCISE

The instructions in the section "Seated Two-Part Deep-Breathing Exercise" also apply to standing two-part deep breathing.

STANDING JOINT RANGE-OF-MOTION EXERCISES

The seated ROM exercises can be adapted to standing exercises. The instructions for teaching the seated ROM exercises in the section "Illustrated Range-of-Motion Instruction" at the end of this chapter apply to both the seated and standing exercises unless otherwise indicated.

Before leading the standing ROM exercises, note the following tips:

- Start with the basic seated warm-ups.
- Review the photographs, teaching instructions, and variations and progression options at the end of this chapter, which apply to both the seated and standing exercises unless otherwise indicated.
- If a participant has difficulty with a standing ROM exercise, he or she can do the corresponding seated exercise.

INSTRUCTIONS FOR GOOD STANDING POSTURE

1. Hands: Relax your hands by your sides or on the back of a chair for support.[a]
2. Hips: Stand erect. Place your hand behind you and feel the curve of your lower back.
3. Feet: Place your feet about hip distance apart, toes pointed forward.
4. Knees: Do not lock your knees; keep them "soft" but not bent ("Ease at the knees").
5. Chest: Take a big breath, and feel your chest lift and expand. Maintain that lifted feeling.
6. Shoulders: Shrug, and then relax your shoulders while maintaining erect posture (see Shoulder Shrugs, exercise 4.17). Repeat as needed.
7. Head and neck: Keep the bottom of your chin parallel with the floor.

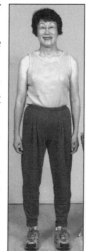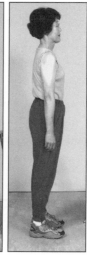

Check each participant for good standing posture.

Visualization: To help maintain good posture, imagine a string attached to the top of your head, pulling gently. Your torso is lengthening with ease.

[a]Suggest that your participants use the chair as a ballet bar. This can be an uplifting image.

From *Exercise for Frail Elders* by E. Best-Martini and K. A. Botenhagen-DiGenova, 2003, Champaign, IL: Human Kinetics.

- Start with either the lower- or upper-body ROM exercises; and do a posture and breathing exercises before the ROM exercises.
- Do the challenger, Standing Mad and Mellow Cat, after participants are comfortable with the other basic standing exercises.

STANDING STRETCHING EXERCISES

The seated stretching exercises can be adapted as standing exercises. Teach standing stretching exercises after the ROM exercises, when your participants are warmed up. Two sets of warm-up stretching exercises for you to choose from appear in table 4.3, "The Minimal Five Stretching Exercises," and table 4.4, "Eight Warm-Up Stretches," both of which are shorter than the comprehensive set of 12 stretching exercises in chapter 7. All the stretching exercises are illustrated and described in chapter 7, which also gives safety tips and variations and progression options for each stretch. You may copy tables 4.3 and 4.4 for use during class.

VARIATIONS AND PROGRESSION

The "Illustrated Range-of-Motion Instruction" section at the end of the chapter gives variations and progression options for each basic warm-up ROM exercise. You have the option of introducing one or more of these exercises after your participants have learned the basic seated exercises. Some participants thrive on regular change. Others, such as those with dementia, may prefer consistency, minimal variation, and slow and steady progress.

In general you can vary a ROM exercise by

- progressing from smaller to larger movements to explore the potential pain-free joint ROM,
- varying the rate (going a little faster or slower),
- varying the rhythm, and
- using music (but keep the movements smooth and not too fast).

For more ideas, see the section "Duration of Warm-Ups" in chapter 8.

The primary progression option is the standing version of an exercise. The benefits of the standing exercises and when the seated version is preferred are discussed in chapter 8.

There are countless ways of varying and progressing an exercise program. When your class is ready for a greater challenge, you can introduce variations of one or more of the basic exercises. For example, if your class particularly enjoys the Seated Shoulder Rotation, you can add a variation such as shoulder rotation with straight-arm circles. You might introduce one new ROM variation each class, each week, or each month. You could introduce one new ROM variation for each target joint. After teaching a variation of an exercise, you can later reintroduce the basic exercise or alternate the basic version and the variation, or you can teach the basic exercise and the variation at the same time. For many other ideas for varying and progressing your class, see chapter 8.

SUMMARY

Participants should always warm up before exercise for 10 minutes at a minimum to ease the transition from rest to exercise. An ideal warm-up for frail elders and adults with special needs includes posture, breathing, ROM, and stretching exercises. This chapter presented guidelines, safety precautions, and teaching instructions for warm-up exercises that enable you to lead a constructive and enjoyable warm-up session.

ILLUSTRATED RANGE-OF-MOTION INSTRUCTION

Exercises 4.1 to 4.6 are lower-body ROM exercises, and exercises 4.7 to 4.24 are for the upper body. The "Exercise and Safety Tips" and "Variations and Progression Options" apply to both seated and standing exercises unless otherwise specified.

SEATED UP-AND-DOWN LEG MARCH

Target Joint   Hips

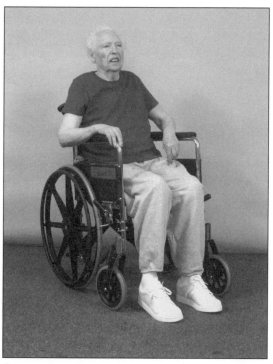

A

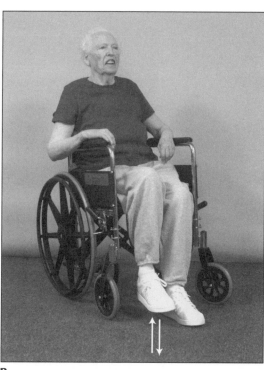

B

START/FINISH POSITION
1. Good seated posture.*
2. Hands in comfortable position.

UPWARD/DOWNWARD MOVEMENT
3. Lift one foot off floor.
4. Then put it back down.
5. Alternate legs (march).
6. Perform three to eight repetitions per leg.

Exercise and Safety Tips
- Lift legs only as high as comfortable while maintaining erect posture.

Variations and Progression Options
- Start by lifting legs slightly, keeping toes on floor. Slowly progress higher.
- Move feet forward and backward while marching.
- Swing arms while marching.
- Perform leg marching between other exercises.
- Standing Up-and-Down Leg March.

*See "Instructions for Good Seated Posture," page 63.

SEATED OUT-AND-IN LEG MARCH

Target Joint   Hips

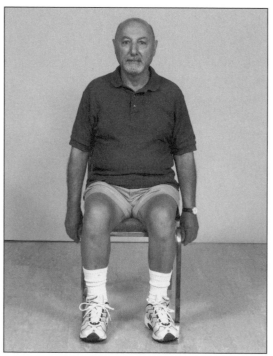

A

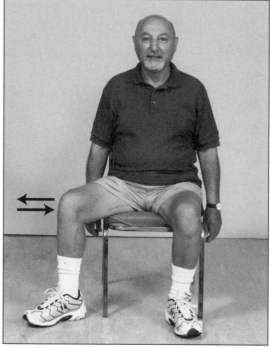

B

START/FINISH POSITION
1. Good seated posture.*
2. Hands in comfortable position.

OUTWARD/INWARD MOVEMENT
3. Lift one leg out to the side.
4. Then move it back to center.
5. Alternate legs (march).
6. Perform three to eight repetitions per leg.

Exercise and Safety Tips
- Keep each foot directly below each knee.

Variations and Progression Options
- Start by lifting legs slightly; progress to higher movements.
- Swing arms while marching.
- Perform leg marching between other exercises.
- Standing Out-and-In Leg March.

*See "Instructions for Good Seated Posture," page 63.

SEATED HIP ROTATION

Target Joint   Hips

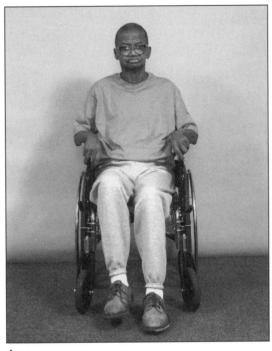

A

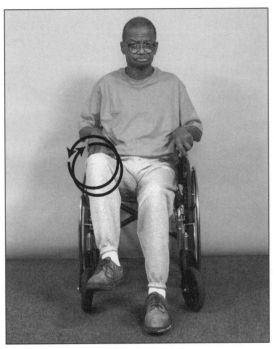

B

START/FINISH POSITION

1. Good seated posture.*
2. Hands in comfortable position.
3. Lift foot 1 to 2 inches (2.5–5 centimeters) off floor.

CIRCULAR MOVEMENT

4. Make circles with one knee in one direction. Move knee up, out, down, and in.
5. Perform three to eight repetitions.
6. Rest foot on floor.
7. Repeat in opposite direction.
8. Repeat steps 3 to 7 with the other leg.

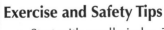

Exercise and Safety Tips

- Start with small circles. The toes do not need to leave the floor at first.

Variations and Progression Options

- Initially, support the rotating leg with one or both hands; progress to unsupported rotations.
- Progress to larger circles. Be creative with circle sizes.
- Lift foot 3 inches (8 centimeters) or more off floor.
- Standing Hip Rotation: Make circles with the foot.

*See "Instructions for Good Seated Posture," page 63.

SEATED BEST FOOT FORWARD AND BACKWARD

Target Joint Knees

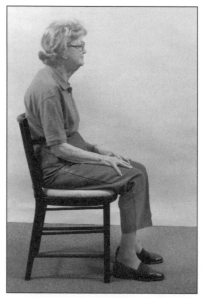 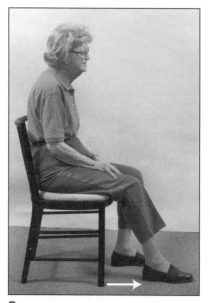 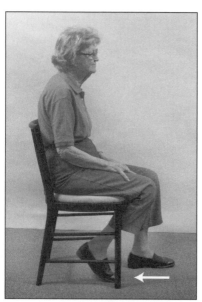

A   B

START/FINISH POSITION

1. Good seated posture.*
2. Hands in comfortable position.

FORWARD/BACKWARD MOVEMENT

3. Step forward with one foot.
4. Then swing foot backward under chair.
5. Perform three to eight repetitions.
6. Repeat with the other leg.

Exercise and Safety Tips

- Modification: If chairs have bars prohibiting legs from going under seat, bring foot back as far as possible.

Variations and Progression Options

- Do a gentle heel tap or toe tap forward.
- Alternate heel tap, then toe tap.
- Standing Best Foot Forward and Backward.

*See "Instructions for Good Seated Posture," page 63.

SEATED TOE POINT AND FLEX

Target Joint   Ankles

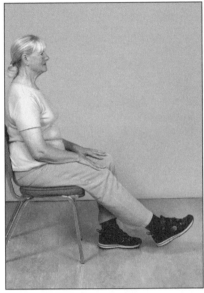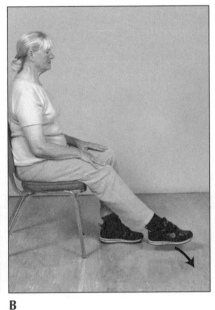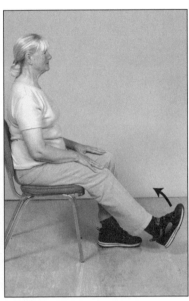

A   **B**

START/FINISH POSITION

1. Good seated posture.*
2. Hands in comfortable position.
3. Slide one foot forward as far as comfortable.
4. Lift same foot 1 to 2 inches (2.5– 5 centimeters) off floor.

DOWNWARD/UPWARD MOVEMENT

5. Point toes and flex ankle.
6. Perform three to eight repetitions.
7. Repeat with the other leg.

Exercise and Safety Tips

- Perform Standing Toe Point and Flex while holding on to a secure support.
- Avoid locking the knee of supporting leg during Standing Toe Point and Flex.

Variations and Progression Options

- Lift foot 3 inches (8 centimeters) or more off floor.
- Standing Toe Point and Flex.

*See "Instructions for Good Seated Posture," page 63.

SEATED ANKLE ROTATIONS

Target Joint   Ankles

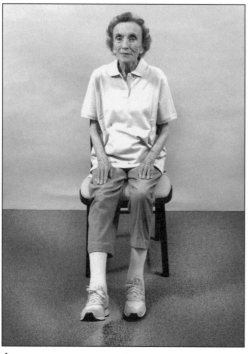

A

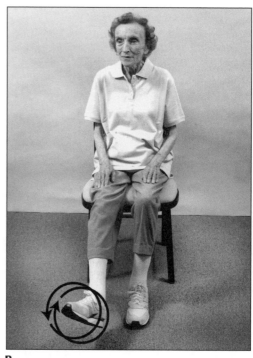

B

START/FINISH POSITION

1. Good seated posture.*
2. Hands in comfortable position.
3. Lift foot 1 to 2 inches (2.5–5 centimeters) off floor.

CIRCULAR MOVEMENT

4. Make circles with toes in one direction. Move toes up, out, down, and in.
5. Perform three to eight repetitions.
6. Repeat in opposite direction.
7. Repeat with the other leg.

Exercise and Safety Tips

- Perform Standing Ankle Rotations while holding on to a secure support.
- Avoid locking the knee of standing leg during Standing Ankle Rotations.

Variations and Progression Options

- Be creative with circle sizes.
- Lift foot 3 inches (8 centimeters) or more off floor.
- Standing Ankle Rotations.

*See "Instructions for Good Seated Posture," page 63.

SEATED MAD AND MELLOW CAT (CHALLENGER)

Target Joint   Spine

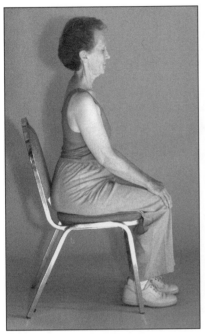 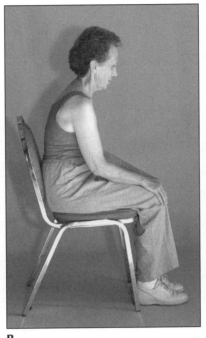 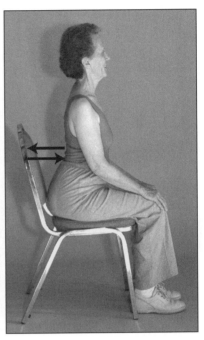

A   B

START/FINISH POSITION

1. Good seated posture.*
2. Hands in comfortable position.

BACKWARD/FORWARD MOVEMENT

3. Press lower back into chair back (mad cat).
4. Come back to neutral position.
5. Gently arch back (mellow cat).
6. Return to neutral position.
7. Perform three to eight repetitions.

Exercise and Safety Tips

- Put hands on hips to feel pelvis moving backward and forward.
- Do not hyperextend the neck in the arched "mellow cat" position. Look forward, not up.

Variations and Progression Options

- Review the natural curve of the spine (see figure 4.2) with participants.
- Visualization: Imagine a string extending from the belly button that when gently pulled makes the back arch. Then press belly button into the back of chair.
- Standing Mad and Mellow Cat (challenger).

*See "Instructions for Good Seated Posture," page 63.

SEATED SIDE REACH

Target Joint   Spine

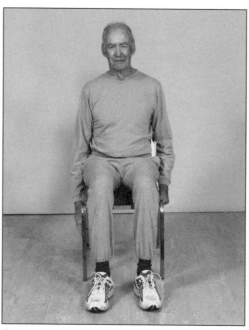

A

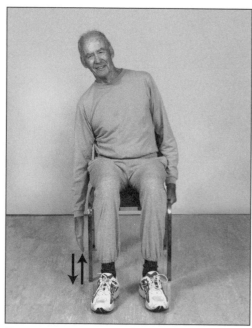

B

START/FINISH POSITION

1. Good seated posture.*
2. Hold side of chair with one hand.
3. Opposite arm straight at side, palm facing in.

DOWNWARD/UPWARD MOVEMENT

4. Lower hand toward floor.
5. Return to starting position.
6. Perform three to eight repetitions.
7. Repeat on the other side.

Exercise and Safety Tips

- The back should be warmed up in a vertical position (as in exercise 4.7 Mad and Mellow Cat, 4.18 Rowing, 4.19 Close the Window) before turning or bending the trunk sideways.
- Hold on to arm or seat of chair for support during Seated Side Reach.
- Do not bend the neck. Keep neck and spine in a neutral position.

Variations and Progression Options

- Reach up with one arm overhead.
- Standing Side Reach.

*See "Instructions for Good Seated Posture," page 63.

SEATED TORSO ROTATION

Target Joint   Spine

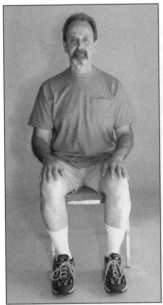 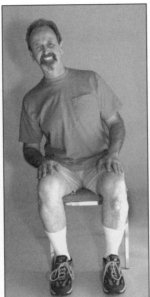 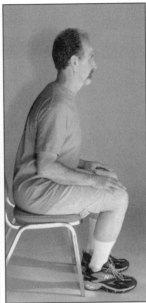 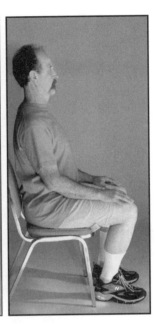

A   **B**

START/FINISH POSITION

1. Good seated posture.*
2. Palms on thighs.

CIRCULAR MOVEMENT

3. Lean to one side.
4. Then lean forward from the hips.
5. Then lean toward the other side (not shown).
6. Then lean slightly backward from the hips.
7. Return to starting position.
8. Perform three to eight repetitions.
9. Repeat in the other direction.

Exercise and Safety Tips

- The back should be warmed up in a vertical position (as in exercise 4.7 Mad and Mellow Cat, 4.18 Rowing, 4.19 Close the Window) before turning or bending the trunk sideways.
- Palms should rest on thighs when leaning forward in Seated Torso Rotation.
- Move head, neck, and spine as one unit.
- Do not hyperextend (overarch) the lower back when leaning backward.

Variations and Progression Options

- Start with small circles; progress to larger ones. Be creative with circle sizes.
- Standing Torso Rotation.

*See "Instructions for Good Seated Posture," page 63.

SEATED TWISTS

Target Joint   Spine

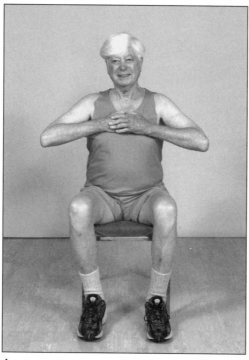

A

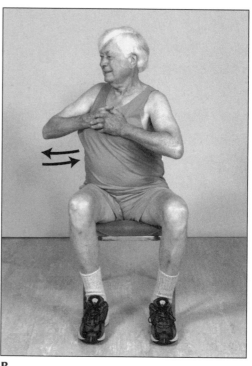

B

START/FINISH POSITION

1. Good seated posture*.
2. Place palms on chest, one hand on top of the other.
3. Elbows out.

TWISTING MOVEMENT

4. Twist the torso, moving one elbow backward, the other forward.
5. Keep shoulders down.
6. Return to starting position.
7. Perform three to eight repetitions.
8. Repeat in the opposite direction.

Exercise and Safety Tips

- Modification: If the back of the chair is in the way, scoot forward in the chair, if this is comfortable.
- Perform twists slowly and smoothly through a comfortable range of motion.
- Do not twist head or neck. Keep the chin aligned with the breastbone.
- Modification: Lower elbows if shoulders or arms get tired.

Variations and Progression Options

- Alternate sides.
- Standing Twists.

*See "Instructions for Good Seated Posture," page 63.

SEATED CHIN TO CHEST ("YES")

Target Joint   Cervical spine (neck)

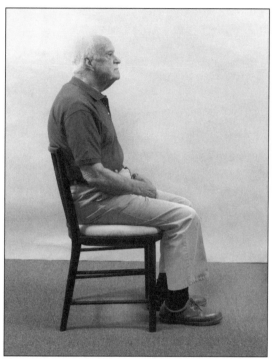

A

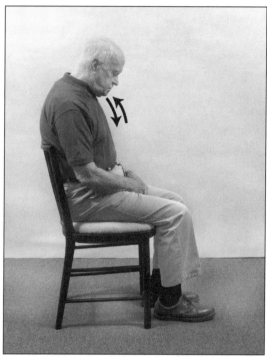

B

START/FINISH POSITION

1. Good seated posture.*
2. Hands in comfortable position.

DOWNWARD/UPWARD MOVEMENT

3. Slowly lower chin toward chest.
4. Slowly lift head back to starting position.
5. Perform three to eight repetitions.

Exercise and Safety Tips

- Do not hyperextend neck; move head slowly.

Variations and Progression Options

- Interlace fingers behind the back and press downward.
- Standing Chin to Chest.

*See "Instructions for Good Seated Posture," page 63.

SEATED CHIN TO SHOULDER

Target Joint   Cervical spine (neck)

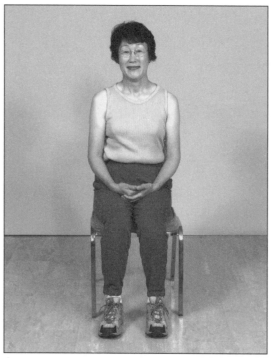

A

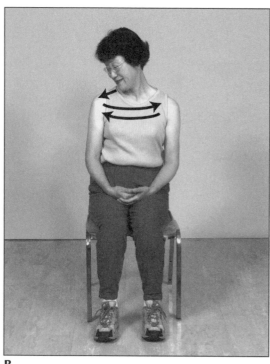

B

START/FINISH POSITION

1. Good seated posture*.
2. Hands in comfortable position.

OUTWARD/INWARD MOVEMENT

3. Lower chin toward shoulder.
4. Rotate chin to chest.
5. Then toward the other shoulder.
6. Rotate back to chest.
7. Then back to the first shoulder.
8. Perform three to eight repetitions.

Exercise and Safety Tips

- Move head slowly and smoothly.

Variations and Progression Options

- Interlace fingers behind the back and press downward.
- Combine Chin to Shoulder with looking at the floor, making a half circle in the front from shoulder to shoulder.
- Standing Chin to Shoulder.

*See "Instructions for Good Seated Posture," page 63.

SEATED ARM SWING

Target Joint Shoulders

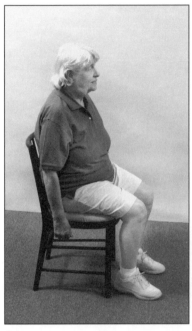

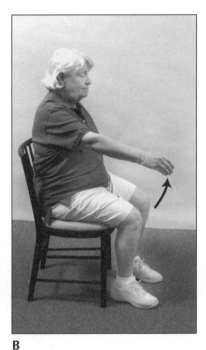

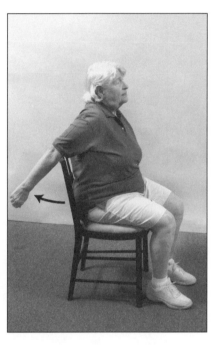

A

B

START/FINISH POSITION

1. Good seated posture.*
2. Hold side of chair on one side.
3. Lean toward opposite side.
4. Free arm straight at side.

FORWARD/BACKWARD MOVEMENT

5. Swing arm forward and backward.
6. Perform three to eight repetitions.
7. Repeat with the other arm.

Exercise and Safety Tips

- Avoid twisting the torso while swinging the arms.
- Gently shake arm before performing Arm Swing to help release residual stiffness so that the arm can swing freely.

Variations and Progression Options

- Use fists or relaxed hands with Arm Swings.
- Use bent or straight arms.
- Standing Arm Swing.

*See "Instructions for Good Seated Posture," page 63.

SEATED BUTTERFLY WINGS

Target Joint   Shoulders

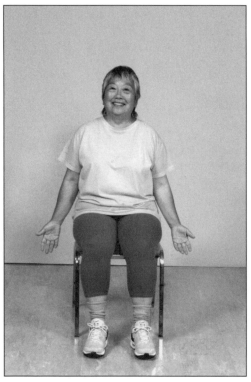

A

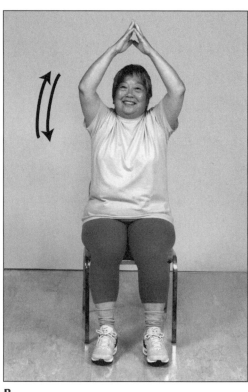

B

START/FINISH POSITION
1. Good seated posture.*
2. Arms straight at sides, palms forward.

UPWARD/DOWNWARD MOVEMENT
3. Raise arms toward ceiling as far as comfortable.
4. Slowly lower arms back to starting position.
5. Perform three to eight repetitions.

Exercise and Safety Tips
- Initially, hold on to a support with one hand and lift one arm at a time during Standing Butterfly Wings. Those without balance problems may progress to lifting both arms simultaneously.

Variations and Progression Options
- Palms up on the upward motion and down on the downward motion.
- Standing Butterfly Wings.

*See "Instructions for Good Seated Posture," page 63.

SEATED SHOULDER ROTATION

Target Joint Shoulders

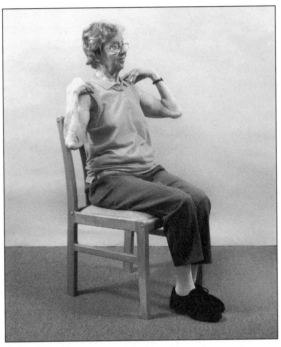

A

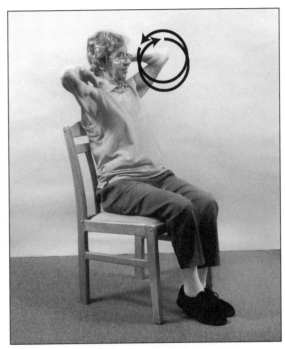

B

START/FINISH POSITION

1. Good seated posture.*
2. Fingertips on shoulders.
3. Elbows out to the sides.

CIRCULAR MOVEMENT

4. Make circles with elbows.
5. Perform three to eight repetitions.
6. Repeat in the other direction.

! Exercise and Safety Tips

- Focus on lifting and opening the chest while rotating shoulders.
- Initially, hold on to a secure support with one hand and rotate one arm at a time during Standing Shoulder Rotations. Those without balance problems may progress to rotating both arms simultaneously.

Variations and Progression Options

- Be creative with circle sizes.
- Rotate straight arms.
- Rotate just the shoulders with arms straight at sides.
- Standing Shoulder Rotation.

*See "Instructions for Good Seated Posture," page 63.

SEATED STIR THE SOUP

Target Joint   Shoulders

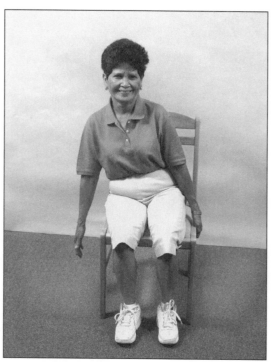

A

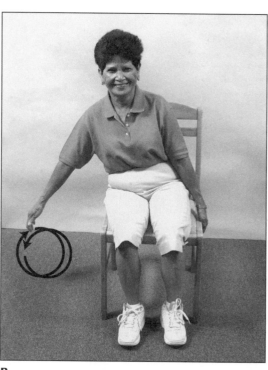

B

START/FINISH POSITION

1. Good seated posture.*
2. Hold side of chair with one arm.
3. Lean toward opposite side.
4. Free arm straight at side.

CIRCULAR MOVEMENT

5. Swing free arm in a circular motion.
6. Perform three to eight repetitions.
7. Repeat in the other direction.
8. Repeat on the other side.

Exercise and Safety Tips

- Hold on to chair seat or arm to prevent falling during Seated Stir the Soup.
- Gently shake arm before performing Stir the Soup to help release residual stiffness so that the arm can freely swing.

Variations and Progression Options

- Be creative with circle sizes.
- Trace different patterns, for example, numbers, letters, or words.
- Standing Stir the Soup.

*See "Instructions for Good Seated Posture," page 63.

SEATED SHOULDER SHRUGS

Target Joint   Shoulders

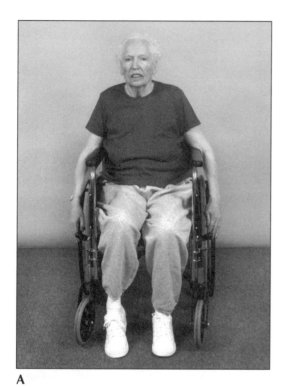

A

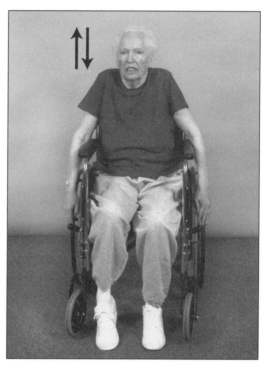

B

START/FINISH POSITION

1. Good seated posture.*
2. Arms straight at sides, palms facing inward.

UPWARD/DOWNWARD MOVEMENT

3. Lift both shoulders toward the ears.
4. Slowly return to starting position.
5. Perform three to eight repetitions.

 Exercise and Safety Tips

- Lower the shoulders smoothly.

Variations and Progression Options

- Start by lifting the shoulders only 1 inch (2.5 centimeters); then lift them progressively higher.
- Standing Shoulder Shrugs.

*See "Instructions for Good Seated Posture," page 63.

SEATED ROWING

Target Joint   Shoulders and elbows

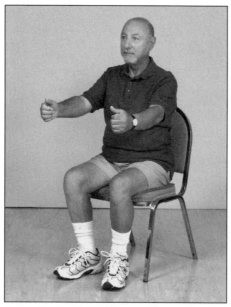

A

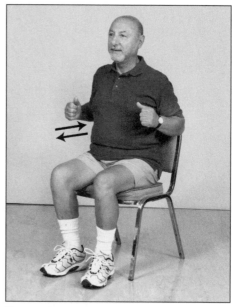

B

START/FINISH POSITION

1. Good seated posture.*
2. Arms straight out in front, slightly below shoulder level.
3. Palms facing inward.

BACKWARD/FORWARD MOVEMENT

4. Pull arms backward in rowing motion.
5. Squeeze shoulder blades together.
6. Perform three to eight repetitions.

Exercise and Safety Tips

- Keep shoulders down.
- Move elbows straight backward, not to the side.
- On the backward rowing motion, gently squeeze shoulder blades together by drawing elbows toward one another behind your back.
- Modification: If it can be done safely, sit toward middle of chair so that elbows clear back of chair.
- Warm up the back by performing 4.18 Rowing and 4.19 Close the Window before the spine ROM exercises, until participants learn 4.7 Mad and Mellow Cat (challenger).

Variations and Progression Options

- Modification: Upper arms can be held lower if participants experience shoulder pain or fatigue or just for variety.
- Row with a narrow grip or a wide grip.
- Row with an underhand grip.
- Standing Rowing.

*See "Instructions for Good Seated Posture," page 63.

SEATED CLOSE THE WINDOW

Target Joint Shoulders and elbows

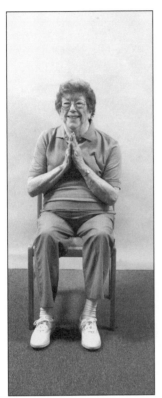

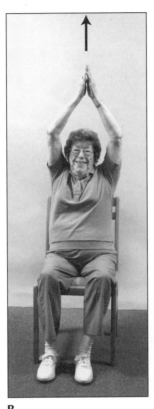

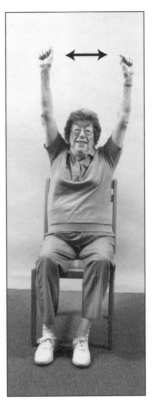

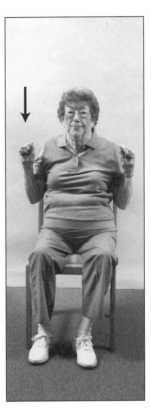

A

B

START/FINISH POSITION

1. Good seated posture.*
2. Hands in prayer position (palms together in front of chest, fingers pointing upward).

UPWARD/DOWNWARD MOVEMENT

3. Lift arms upward as far as comfortable.
4. Open hands, grasp imaginary window frame.
5. Pull down the window.
6. Return to starting position.
7. Perform three to eight repetitions.

Exercise and Safety Tips

- Those recovering from stroke can usually move through a greater ROM on the affected side by clasping their hands instead of pressing palms together.
- Warm up the back by performing 4.18 Rowing and 4.19 Close the Window before the spine ROM exercises, until participants learn 4.7 Mad and Mellow Cat (challenger).

Variations and Progression Options

- Try to put elbows in back pockets (pressing elbows downward and backward) when closing the imaginary window.
- Standing Close the Window.

*See "Instructions for Good Seated Posture," page 63.

SEATED WRIST FLEXION AND EXTENSION

Target Joint   Wrists

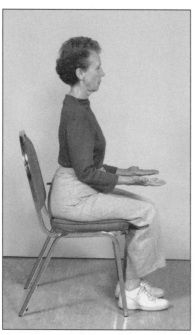

A

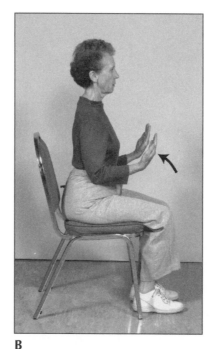

B

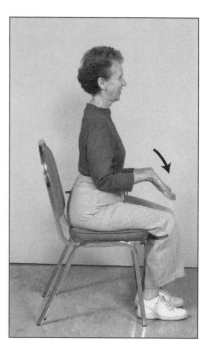

START/FINISH POSITION

1. Good seated posture.*
2. Upper arms by sides.
3. Forearms parallel with lap, palms up.

UPWARD/DOWNWARD MOVEMENT

4. Flex wrists.
5. Extend wrists.
6. Perform three to eight repetitions.

Exercise and Safety Tips

*   Modification: If arms get tired at a 90-degree angle, rest arms by sides and continue flexing and extending.

Variations and Progression Options

*   Palms down.
*   Hold arms in different positions, from straight overhead to straight at the sides.
*   Standing Wrist Flexion and Extension.

*See "Instructions for Good Seated Posture," page 63.

SEATED WRIST ROTATIONS

Target Joint Wrists

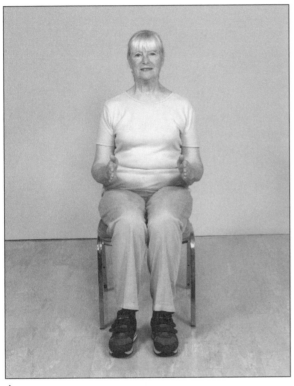

A

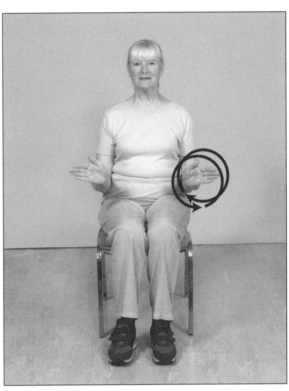

B

START/FINISH POSITION

1. Good seated posture.*
2. Upper arms by sides.
3. Forearms parallel with lap.
4. Palms facing inward.

CIRCULAR MOVEMENT

5. Make circles with wrist in one direction. Move wrists up, out, down, and in.
6. Perform three to eight repetitions.
7. Repeat in opposite direction.

Exercise and Safety Tips

- Modification: If arms get tired at a 90-degree angle, rest arms by sides and continue wrist rotations.

Variations and Progression Options

- Be creative with circle sizes.
- Hold arms in different positions, from straight overhead to straight at the sides.
- Standing Wrist Rotations.

*See "Instructions for Good Seated Posture," page 63.

SEATED HANDS OPEN AND CLOSED

Target Joint Fingers

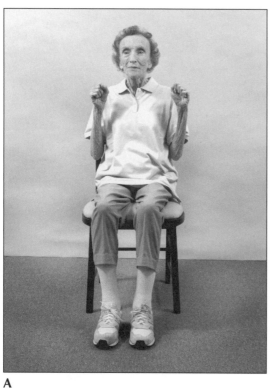

A

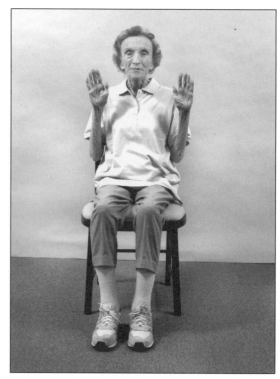

B

START/FINISH POSITION

1. Good seated posture.*
2. Arms in "stick 'em up" position (palms facing forward near shoulders), elbows by sides.
3. Make fists.

OUTWARD/INWARD MOVEMENT

4. Open fists.
5. Close fists.
6. Perform three to eight repetitions.

Exercise and Safety Tips

- Remind those with difficulty moving their hands to go at their own pace and stay within their pain-free range of motion.

Variations and Progression Options

- Open and close hands randomly in different places, like fireworks exploding throughout the sky.
- Standing Hands Open and Closed.

*See "Instructions for Good Seated Posture," page 63.

SEATED SUN RAYS

Target Joint   Fingers

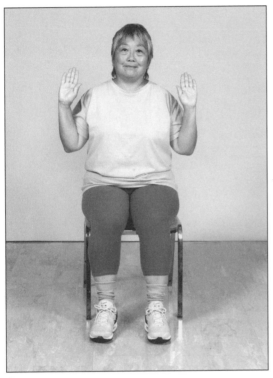

A

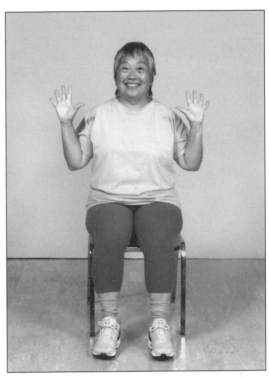

B

START/FINISH POSITION

1. Good seated posture*.
2. Arms in "stick 'em up" position (palms facing forward near shoulders), elbows by sides.
3. Fingers together.

OUTWARD/INWARD MOVEMENT

4. Spread fingers apart.
5. Then move them back together.
6. Perform three to eight repetitions.

Exercise and Safety Tips

- Remind those with difficulty moving their hands to go at their own pace and stay within their pain-free range of motion.

Variations and Progression Options

- Move hands up and down while spreading fingers, like rays of the rising and setting sun.
- Standing Sun Rays.

*See "Instructions for Good Seated Posture," page 63.

SEATED PIANO PLAYING

Target Joint   Fingers

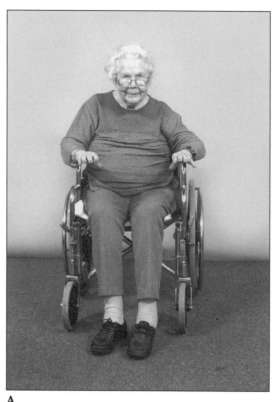

A

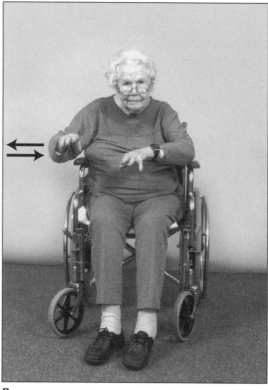

B

START/FINISH POSITION

1. Good seated posture.*
2. Upper arms by sides.
3. Forearms parallel with lap, palms down.

OUTWARD/INWARD MOVEMENT

4. Move fingers and arms as if playing a piano.
5. Perform three to eight repetitions.

Exercise and Safety Tips

- Remind those with difficulty moving their hands to go at their own pace and stay within their pain-free range of motion.
- Modification: If arms get tired at a 90-degree angle, lower arms to lap and continue Seated Piano Playing.

Variations and Progression Options

- Play with a wider "keyboard."
- Standing Piano Playing.

*See "Instructions for Good Seated Posture," page 63.

CHAPTER 5

Aerobic Training for Cardiovascular Endurance

Janie Clark*

Aerobic exercise (moderate-intensity activity involving large muscle groups using oxygen-supplied energy) is done to increase *cardiovascular endurance* (also known as *aerobic fitness*, one's ability to take in, transport, and utilize oxygen). Effective aerobic training produces significant improvements in *cardiovascular* (involving the heart and circulatory system) health.

There are five keys to conducting a successful aerobic exercise program for elderly fitness participants: individualization, proper integration of aerobic-training variables, inclusion of essential exercise-session components, safety awareness, and creativity. This chapter provides guidance in all these important areas.

• **Individualization.** Elderly participants differ in health and fitness status, skill level, and training tolerance. In this chapter, you will learn how to help your aerobics participants pace themselves effectively and how to adapt your program for those who need modifications in order to perform well.

• **Integration of training variables.** Factors such as intensity, frequency, and duration must be set in a way that permits gradual, progressive training. Using the guidelines provided in this chapter, start with the lower-body movements of the basic seated aerobic exercises. You will learn to add upper-body movements safely and to help certain participants perform the basic standing aerobic exercises. The seated and standing exercises are designed to be taught at the same time so that your exercise class can accommodate individuals of various performance abilities.

• **Inclusion of essential components.** Your aerobic exercise class should feature three phases: an initial warm-up period of light movement and stretches (see chapter 4), the aerobic exercises, and a cool-down period of light movement followed by stretching (see chapter 7). Table 5.1 provides an overview. A good way to include resistance training in the class is to complete the three phases described above, followed by resistance training and another cool-down period. Warm-up and cool-down periods include activities performed with aerobically produced energy. Indeed, they may include many of the same exercises as the main aerobic-training component itself. However, movements during the aerobic phase of the workout should be performed more energetically and for a longer duration (Clark 1998).

• **Safety awareness.** In fitness programming for frail elders and adults with special needs, nothing is more important than safety. Following the detailed safety guidelines provided in this chapter helps keep your aerobics participants injury-free. In your day-to-day work, always keep in mind this important advice: "Generally, older persons are more fragile, more susceptible to orthopedic injury and possible cardiovascular problems. Therefore, [aerobic] exercise prescription should emphasize low-moderate intensity exercise, low-impact activity,

*Janie Clark, MA, is an exercise physiologist and is president of the American Senior Fitness Association, New Smyrna Beach, Florida.

TABLE 5.1	COMPONENTS OF AN AEROBIC EXERCISE SESSION FOR OLDER ADULTS	
Component	**Includes these exercises**	**Duration**
Warm-up (see chapter 4)	Posture awareness Deep breathing Range-of-motion exercises Easy-paced activities such as slow walking Mild stretching	10–15 minutes
Aerobic exercise	Low- to moderate-intensity rhythmic work using large muscle groups	Time permitting, build up to 30–60 minutes (depending on intensity)
Cool-down (see chapter 7)	Low-intensity aerobic exercises Light, limbering ROM movements Sustained stretching Relaxation	10–15 minutes

starting slowly, and gradually progressing in duration and frequency" (Swart, Pollock, and Brechue 1996, 9).

• **Creativity.** Technical programming criteria pertain to the science of aerobic training. Creativity, however, concerns the *art* of aerobic training. The lively nature of aerobic exercise affords participants extraordinary opportunities to enjoy movement to music in a stimulating, motivational environment that promotes continued participation. This chapter provides numerous suggestions on how to incorporate music, variety, and fun into your aerobic exercise program.

SAFETY PRECAUTIONS FOR AEROBIC TRAINING

Aerobic training can be safe for older adults if appropriate training guidelines and precautions are observed. The following "General Safety Precautions Checklist for Aerobics" and "Specific Safety Precautions for Those With Special Needs" help you lead safe aerobics and keep your participants injury-free. You may photocopy the "General Safety Precautions Checklist" for aerobics and the "Safety Guidelines Checklist" in chapter 2.

General Safety Precautions Checklist for Aerobics

❑ It is critical that people who lead aerobic training for frail elderly adults hold both CPR and first-aid certification.

❑ Before initiating aerobic training, review any special do's and don'ts that the physician has written on the medical clearance form.

❑ Aerobics participants should wear sturdy shoes with adequate arch support and ample cushioning.

❑ Seated participants should be able to place their backs securely against the backs of their chairs or wheelchairs while keeping their feet flat on the floor. If not, correct their positioning with pillows or platforms.

❑ Remind seated and standing participants to maintain good posture.

❑ Participants with blindness, extreme frailty, or balance problems that place them at risk of falling should perform only seated aerobic exercise.

From *Exercise for Frail Elders* by E. Best-Martini and K. A. Botenhagen-DiGenova, 2003, Champaign, IL: Human Kinetics.

❑ Perform only *low-impact activity* (exercise that does not significantly jar the joints).

❑ Demonstrate all aerobic exercises in a controlled manner at a moderate speed.

❑ Do not use weights or any type of resistive equipment during aerobic training. Nonresistive accessories, such as scarves, may be used.

❑ Avoid jerking or slinging motions of the limbs. Encourage smooth, rhythmic movement.

❑ Don't overdo it. Aerobic exercise should energize participants, not exhaust them.

❑ Remind participants to pace themselves.

❑ Instruct your participants to never hold their breath during aerobic exercise. They need a steady supply of oxygen to produce the energy necessary to sustain continuous movement. Have participants sing along with familiar workout tunes. Counting aloud is another good practice. During the prolonged performance of a single exercise, ask individuals open-ended questions. Participants cannot hold their breath when vocalizing.

❑ In addition to using ratings of perceived exertion (RPE; discussed later in this chapter), always observe your participants closely during aerobic exercise. Stay alert for warning signs such as labored breathing.

❑ Even more than other forms of exercise, aerobic training requires thorough warm-up and cool-down periods, especially for elderly participants. Most cardiac complications that occur during exercise arise at the beginning or end of workouts. Warming up is vital because the heart and circulation need sufficient transition time to slowly accommodate the increased oxygen demands of aerobic exercise. The cool-down prevents potentially dangerous blood pooling in the lower extremities and lowers the risk of *arrhythmia* (abnormal heart rhythm). In aerobic training, warm up and cool down for a minimum of 10 to 15 minutes. Begin the aerobics-class warm-up with low-intensity limbering movements, proceed to light calisthenics and other easy-paced activities such as slow walking, and conclude with mild stretching. Begin the aerobics-class cool-down with low-intensity aerobic exercise, proceed to lighter limbering movements, and conclude with sustained stretches (American Senior Fitness Association 2003c).

❑ In aerobics classes for frail elderly participants, an entirely noncompetitive atmosphere should be maintained.

❑ Because aerobic exercise promotes sweating, it is important to provide participants with opportunities for fluid replacement. Make water available before, during, and after aerobic training.

❑ Participants should not perform aerobic exercise with an elevated body temperature. They should wait until body temperature has been normal again for 24 hours and then gradually resume activity.

❑ When returning from a layoff, participants should resume aerobic training at a rating of perceived exertion of 12 or less, then gradually build back up to an RPE of 12 to 14.

From *Exercise for Frail Elders* by E. Best-Martini and K. A. Botenhagen-DiGenova, 2003, Champaign, IL: Human Kinetics.

95

Specific Safety Precautions for Those With Special Needs

In serving elders with special needs, keep in mind that aerobic exercise engages not only the cardiovascular system but also the pulmonary, nervous, and musculoskeletal systems. Follow the appropriate specific safety precautions when leading aerobic training for those special needs.

Alzheimer's Disease and Related Dementias

- Participants with cognitive impairments may not perform well when asked to learn numerous dance-exercise moves; an aerobics program based mainly on walking can be especially beneficial for them (American Senior Fitness Association 2003a).

- Since confused or disoriented participants may not be able to rate their exertion reliably, your constant and unfailing observation is essential.

Arthritis

- Thorough warm-up and cool-down periods are especially critical for aerobics participants with arthritis. Their joints need extra time to prepare for and recover from extended periods of continuous activity.

- If a participant experiences a flare-up of arthritis, modify or suspend exercise activity, but aerobic training should be resumed (in a gradual manner, if necessary) as soon as the participant is able (Caldwell 1996).

Cerebrovascular Accident (Stroke)

- See also the safety precautions for those with coronary artery disease (heart disease).

- Providing clear instructions is extremely important to aerobics participants who have experienced stroke. If a participant has paralysis on the right side, focus on leading exercises mainly by demonstration, using few verbal instructions. If there is paralysis on the left side, rely more on verbal instructions, using fewer gestures (American Senior Fitness Association 2003c).

Chronic Obstructive Pulmonary Disease

- Thorough warm-up and cool-down periods are especially critical for aerobics participants with COPD. Their lungs and cardiovascular systems need extra time to adapt to changes in exertion level.

- All older adults should perform only modest amounts of overhead arm work, but such movements should be even more limited for those who have COPD. In people with COPD, excessive overhead work unduly raises *ventilatory demand* (the amount of air that must be breathed in and out to satisfy the body's need for oxygen and to dispose of carbon dioxide waste).

- Here are three different methods that can help prevent breathlessness during aerobic training:

  1. Alternate energetic training periods with easy training periods during the workout. For example, work briskly for five minutes, then lightly for five minutes, and continue alternating. Use longer easy periods if needed.

  2. Accumulate the desired duration by performing short bouts of exercise throughout the day (see "Training Duration" later in this chapter).

  3. Work at an intensity near the lower end of the desirable range (an RPE of 12 instead of an RPE from 12 to 14), but for a longer duration (American Senior Fitness Association 2003c).

- A participant who has an inhaler should use it according to the physician's instructions to prevent or minimize exercise-induced asthma.

Coronary Artery Disease (Heart Disease)

- Thorough warm-up and cool-down periods are especially critical for aerobics participants with heart disease. Their cardiovascular systems need extra time to adapt to changes in exertion level.

- All older adults should perform only modest amounts of overhead arm work, but such movements should be even more limited for those who have heart disease. Excessive overhead work can raise blood pressure.

- It is a good practice to monitor pre- and postexercise blood pressure and pulse rate.

DEPRESSION

- Because aerobic exercise stimulates the brain to release hormones that foster a sense of well-being, it can be an extremely useful tool in combating depression (Caldwell 1996).
- Strive to make your aerobics class an enjoyable event that participants always look forward to. It is *regular* training that significantly reduces depression.

DIABETES

- Keep in mind that many people with diabetes also develop heart disease. See also the precautions for those with coronary artery disease.
- Since weight loss can help control diabetes, appropriate long-term aerobic training can be valuable.
- Be vigilant in watching for symptoms of diabetic emergency. Keep on hand simple carbohydrates that are readily digestible, such as sugar, candy, or fruit juice.
- Make sure that participants with diabetes wear proper socks and shoes. Take special care to avoid injuries to the feet. In people with diabetes, small injuries tend to develop more quickly into serious problems and complications, especially when nerves are diseased or circulation is restricted. At the first sign of any foot problem (e.g., a minor cut), seek medical care (American Senior Fitness Association 2003c).

HYPERTENSION

- See also the precautions for coronary artery disease.
- Since weight loss helps reduce or control blood pressure, appropriate long-term aerobic training can be valuable.

OSTEOPOROSIS

- When symptoms are minor, walking or low-impact aerobic dance can be undertaken as tolerated and may be beneficial in managing the disease.
- An ambulatory participant can combine seated and standing activities during a single aerobics session to perform successfully.
- When osteoporosis is advanced, standing exercise may not be safe because of increased risk for falling and fracture. In that case, the participant should do only seated aerobics.

PARKINSON'S DISEASE AND MULTIPLE SCLEROSIS

- The aerobics participant with Parkinson's disease or multiple sclerosis may need extra reminders and encouragement to maintain optimal posture.
- Many people with Parkinson's disease or multiple sclerosis are at high risk of falling. Ask the physician if an affected frail elderly individual should remain on an all-seated aerobic exercise program (American Senior Fitness Association 2003a).

SENSORY LOSSES

- Standing dance activities to music can be enjoyable and beneficial for people with visual impairments. However, it is safer to use such activities to promote pleasure, creativity, and range of motion than as a means of aerobic conditioning. Structured aerobic training should be done in a seated position by people with visual impairments.
- Provide clear and effective voice cues to people with visual impairment.
- Provide clear and effective demonstration cues to people with hearing loss. Appropriate visual gestures enhance the participant's ability to follow verbal instructions.
- Consider using instrumental music, since it may be easier for participants with hearing loss to follow directions when your voice does not have to compete with vocals in the music (American Senior Fitness Association 2003a; Clark 1992).

GUIDELINES FOR AEROBIC TRAINING

Several prominent organizations have developed guidelines for safe and effective aerobic training, including the American Senior Fitness Association, the American Heart Association, the American College of Sports Medicine, and the Centers for Disease Control and Prevention. Table 5.2 provides a conservative synthesis of their guidelines, specifically adapted by the American Senior Fitness Association to be appropriate for frail elderly participants. The basic seated and standing aerobic exercises in this chapter are based on these well-researched guidelines. You may make a copy of table 5.2 for easy reference.

TABLE 5.2	GENERAL AEROBIC-TRAINING GUIDELINES FOR OLDER ADULTS
Exercise selection	At least one safe, low-impact exercise (such as walking) that uses large muscle groups or a combination of such exercises (such as the aerobic program in this chapter)
Exercise sequence	As desired and well tolerated
Training intensity	12–14 on the RPE scale ("somewhat hard")
Training frequency	3–5 days per week
Training duration	Time permitting, build up to 30 continuous minutes of low to moderate work or up to 60 minutes when only very low intensity work is tolerated. If needed, the desired duration can be accumulated by performing short bouts of activity.
Training range of motion	Through the full, pain-free range of joint movement without hyperextending (overreaching), except when a reduced range is necessary to control intensity
Training speed	A moderate speed that facilitates rhythmic, controlled movement through a broad range of motion
Number of repetitions	As desired and well tolerated
Rest periods	Rest breaks as necessary, with continuous movement or easy, light activity when possible rather than complete cessation of movement
Progression and maintenance	Gradual, conservative increases in frequency and duration (and, to a lesser extent, intensity); continued long-term training after the desired health and fitness level is reached

From *Exercise for Frail Elders* by E. Best-Martini and K. A. Botenhagen-DiGenova, 2003, Champaign, IL: Human Kinetics.

Even more than other forms of exercise, participation in aerobic training calls for medical approval. Dr. Michael L. Pollock, writing with colleagues (Swart, Pollock, and Brechue 1996, 16), stated that aerobic exercise for elderly participants "should be individualized and should include specific recommendations for frequency, intensity, duration and mode of training, based on the results of exercise testing and any limitations that may be imposed by the musculoskeletal system or disease/health status." Your participant's physician is familiar with exercise testing procedures and can administer any indicated laboratory tests during the medical clearance process. Once participants have secured medical approval for a gentle program of aerobic conditioning, they can work productively within a set of general guidelines—so long as only activities that prove to be well tolerated are pursued (Clark 2003).

The following sections offer guidelines to prevent injury and maximize the benefits of aerobic training for frail elders and adults with special needs.

EXERCISE SELECTION

The exercise program in this chapter includes 10 basic aerobic exercises that contribute to cardiovascular health and endurance. These exercises are safe and appropriate for frail elders and adults with special needs who have medical clearance. Teach the basic seated lower-body movements first. Progress to incorporating the corresponding upper-body movements. Participants who are able to do so safely can progress further to standing aerobic exercises.

Other forms of low-impact aerobic conditioning, such as stationary cycling, rowing, treadmill walking, and water activities, also can be considered. Rotating different types of aerobic exercise engages different muscle groups, decreases the odds for overuse injuries, and can increase exercise adherence. In all cases, participants' safety should be the first consideration. Therefore, all risks must be anticipated and eliminated in advance (Swart, Pollock, and Brechue 1996).

EXERCISE SEQUENCE

If the aerobic training session follows a proper warm-up period, the aerobic exercises in this chapter can be performed in any order that you deem practical. These are some important considerations:

1. Many people perform their best when the graph of energy expenditure during aerobic exercise is bell-shaped. That is, begin with easier, lighter movements. Gradually build up to more and more demanding movements. After "peak" moves (the most energetic of your workout), move back through less and less demanding exercises until you return to the easiest and lightest.

2. Depending on how well participants tolerate the bell-shaped model just described, it may be necessary to pace them by interspersing easy, light moves throughout the aerobics session. Individual participants should always be encouraged to pace themselves as needed during group aerobic training.

TRAINING INTENSITY

Aerobic exercise intensity (how hard to work) must be controlled for two important reasons:

1. Excessive intensity can lead to cardiovascular complications and musculoskeletal injuries.

2. On the other hand, insufficient intensity does not produce the desired training effects (Swart, Pollock, and Brechue 1996).

How can you help participants find that middle ground where their aerobic efforts are both safe and effective? A useful tool for monitoring aerobic exercise intensity is the Borg rating of perceived exertion (RPE) scale (Borg 1998; see figure 5.1). This scale, based on the participant's feelings of fatigue, provides a subjective guide to his or her response to exercise. Generally, a rating of from 12 to 14 ("somewhat hard") is a suitable range for improving health and fitness in the elderly (Pollock et al. 1994). Ask

6	No exertion at all
7	
8	Extremely light
9	Very light
10	
11	Light
12	
13	Somewhat hard
14	
15	Hard (heavy)
16	
17	Very hard
18	
19	Extremely hard
20	Maximal exertion

Borg RPE scale
© Gunnar Borg, 1970, 1985, 1994, 1998

FIGURE 5.1 The rating of perceived exertion (RPE) scale is a subjective method of monitoring intensity level. To understand the RPE scale and its administration, see Borg (1998).

Reprinted, by permission, from G. Borg, 1998, *Borg's Perceived Exertion and Pain Scales* (Champaign, IL: Human Kinetics), 47.

your participants to express their RPE frequently during aerobic training. With frail elderly participants, especially beginners, it is not unreasonable to check every few minutes.

Throughout the aerobic exercise session, participants should work at a pace that allows them to breathe naturally and never feel uncomfortably short of breath. They should be able to talk normally at all times. Otherwise, the intensity level is too high and needs to be reduced. When conducting aerobic exercise for frail elderly participants, you should constantly aim for low to moderate effort.

TRAINING FREQUENCY

Initially, schedule aerobic training three days per week (on nonconsecutive days, if possible). After your participants respond favorably to aerobic training for several months, increase the frequency to four and then five times per week. This increases the chance of your participants' making it to class at least three times per week. Encourage beginners to your class to start with three days and slowly progress to five.

TRAINING DURATION

A sound approach is to schedule 10- to 15-minute aerobic exercise sessions initially (preceded and followed by 10- to 15-minute periods of light movement and stretching). Try increasing aerobic exercise duration by 5-minute increments every four weeks until participants are performing sustained aerobic exercise for 30 minutes or longer (Swart, Pollock, and Brechue 1996). Encourage beginners to your class to pace themselves as necessary and to progress slowly to performing the entire aerobics routine.

Especially at first, duration can be limited by the participant's tolerance. In that case, rest breaks can be interspersed with aerobic exercise periods to accumulate the recommended exercise time. In other words, the recommended duration can be accumulated either in one exercise session or during several short activity bouts throughout the day. (If such bouts are undertaken in separate sessions, take care to include adequate warm-up and cool-down periods.) This type of intermittent aerobic activity produces health benefits similar to those achieved through continuous movement (Coleman et al. 1999; DeBusk et al. 1990; Pate et al. 1995; Swart, Pollock, and Brechue 1996).

If time constraints prevent you from scheduling classes that include 30 minutes of aerobic exercise, aerobics sessions from 15 to 20 minutes in duration are also productive. However, there is a good reason to try to extend aerobic training to 30 minutes for frail elderly participants when possible: For a given quantity of work, the intensity and duration of training are inversely related. That is, activities of lower intensity and longer duration provide the same benefits as those of higher intensity and shorter duration. Since low- to moderate-intensity exercise is preferred for frail elderly populations, a longer duration of up to 30 minutes helps to ensure that participants reap maximum benefits. In fact, people who can tolerate only very low intensity work can benefit from durations of up to 60 minutes (Swart, Pollock, and Brechue 1996).

TRAINING RANGE OF MOTION

Using fuller ranges of motion (such as higher limb elevations) increases intensity level, whereas using limited ranges reduces it. Fuller ranges contribute more toward preserving mobility than do limited ranges. As participants become fatigued during the course of an aerobic exercise session, they may need to decrease range in order to maintain an RPE of 12 to 14 ("somewhat hard," not "hard" or "very hard"). Otherwise, remind them to work through their full, pain-free range of joint movement without hyperextending their joints (Clark 1992).

TRAINING SPEED

Aerobic movement that is too fast can cause orthopedic injuries, raise intensity too high, and take the pleasure out of training. Set a rhythmic pace that allows controlled movement through a broad range of motion. If your participants begin flinging their limbs or their form is compromised (e.g., only partial arm reaches when you are teaching fully extended reaches), you should reduce speed. Remind participants that their individual ranges of motion vary and to stay within their pain-free range of motion. Well-chosen music during the aerobic exercise session can help set an appropriate pace while adding fun to your workout. Choose musical numbers that your participants enjoy and perhaps remember fondly. These are some good styles:

- Marches
- Show tunes
- Country
- Gospel
- Ragtime
- Old standards
- Swing

- Popular symphony overtures
- Light pop
- Easy listening
- Calypso and tropical sounds
- Music from around the world

To promote participation and prevent discomfort among participants, always keep the volume conservative.

Many instructors find it convenient to establish the right pace by using tunes with a specific number of beats per minute (BPM). Commercial exercise music marketers offer audiotapes and compact discs labeled with the BPM (see "Suggested Resources" near the end of this book). For active, independent-living older adults, a tempo from 120 to 140 BPM is viable during aerobic exercise. For frail elderly participants, try a range from 110 to 130 BPM or even slower (American Senior Fitness Association 2003b).

Whether or not you select music based on its BPM, remember that the beat of your music must facilitate the three major goals discussed earlier:

1. Rhythmic activity
2. Controlled movement
3. Broad ranges of motion

NUMBER OF REPETITIONS

In aerobic exercise, there is no strict rule for when to change from one exercise to the next. Indeed, participants can obtain aerobic benefits simply by performing a single aerobic activity (such as walking, cycling, or rowing) at the recommended intensity and duration for the entire exercise session. Therefore, the rate at which you change from one exercise to another should depend on the characteristics of your exercise group. These are some important considerations:

1. Changing too quickly from one aerobic exercise to the next can overwhelm elderly participants, especially beginners. They should do enough repetitions to master the movement and to experience a sense of confidence in performing it before moving on. Ensuring that participants can follow your workout successfully encourages their continued attendance.

2. As participants perfect their skills, you can change moves more frequently. Varying the aerobic exercises promotes several benefits:

- Decreased risk of overuse injury
- Better conditioning of joints and muscles by working them through different angles
- Improved coordination
- Mental stimulation
- Discouraging boredom and increasing interest and enjoyment

3. You can perform a specific exercise, proceed through a series of other moves, and then repeat the original exercise or a variation of it. In fact, you can return to favorite moves often during any single workout session.

REST PERIODS

Elderly aerobics participants should be taught and often reminded to pace themselves as needed throughout the exercise session. At times, participants (beginners especially) may feel the need to cease movement completely. However, as they grow stronger, encourage them to pace themselves by simply slowing down or substituting lighter, easier movements for a while when they feel tired. Sustaining continuous activity in this way can help build endurance.

Keep in mind that some frail elders tolerate aerobic exercise best when it is measured out in short (5- to 10-minute) bouts of activity throughout the day, as long as they accumulate the total recommended duration.

OTHER TRAINING TECHNIQUES

Here is the simplest way to use the exercises in this chapter to lead your initial aerobic workouts:

1. First follow the given order of the exercises. Make the whole sequence last half the desired duration of your aerobics session, and plan the duration of each exercise accordingly. For example, for a 20-minute aerobics session using 10 exercises, perform each exercise for 1 minute for a subtotal of 10 minutes.

2. Then reverse the given order of the exercises, taking the same length of time for each movement. Teaching the given order followed by the reversed order results in an aerobics session of the desired duration with higher-intensity exercises at midpoint and easier exercises at the beginning and end. With practice and experience, you will learn to vary the exercise sequences while maintaining the appropriate intensity throughout your aerobics class.

Develop exercise patterns and combinations, like these:

1. Combine two single exercises into an exercise pattern. For example, perform four Alternate Toe Touches to Front (exercise 5.4), then four Alternate Heel Touches to Front (exercise 5.5), and continue repeating the pattern.

2. When the first pattern has been mastered, teach participants a new pattern. For example, perform four Alternate Toe Touches to Sides (exercise 5.6), then four Alternate Heel Touches to Sides (exercise 5.7), and continue repeating that pattern.

3. When two patterns have been mastered, teach participants a combination of the two: four Alternate Toe Touches to Front, four Alternate Heel Touches to Front, four Alternate Toe Touches to Sides, and four Alternate Heel Touches to Sides. Repeat the combination for as long as desired.

When each exercise also includes its own specific arm moves, such patterns and combinations of patterns create an appealing dance atmosphere—especially if accompanied by music. Developing numerous patterns and combinations adds variety and excitement to your aerobics class. Also, you can recycle your participants' favorite patterns and combinations by performing them to new musical selections.

Supplement the exercises in this chapter with additional aerobic movements that are consistent with your participants' performance ability. Develop your own new exercises by mixing and matching basic lower-body movements with various upper-body movements. For ideas, see "Developing New Aerobic Exercises" on the next page. Achieve even more variety by combining your new exercises into patterns and combinations as described earlier. The variety of your aerobic workouts is limited only by your creativity.

When changing from one aerobic exercise to another, cue your participants clearly and well in advance. Initially, conduct smooth transitions by asking your participants to walk in place briefly after each exercise while you demonstrate the next one for them. This method helps ensure their continuous movement throughout the aerobic workout. As you become more expert at cuing and as your participants grow familiar with the exercises, they will be able to move directly from one exercise to another.

DEVELOPING NEW AEROBIC EXERCISES

Create new moves by mixing and matching the arm movements given below with the leg movements of exercises 5.1 to 5.10 (either seated or standing). All these arm movements are compatible with exercise 5.2 (walking in place). Identify other good match-ups by trying different arm and leg moves together outside of class. Then teach new combinations that work well to your participants during class.

Alternately snap fingers, then clap hands together.

Alternately slap front thighs lightly, then clap hands together.

Reach with both arms in any direction (up, down, front, or out to each side).

Alternately reach with both arms in one direction, then another (for example, front and then out to the sides).

Punch with both arms in any direction (up, down, front, or out to each side).

Alternately punch with both arms in one direction, then another (for example, up and then down).

Push with both hands in any direction (up, down, front, or out to each side).

Alternately push with both hands in one direction, then another (for example, up and then front).

Fly like a bird (gently simulate a bird flapping its wings).

Be a movie reviewer (alternately turn thumbs up, then thumbs down).

Be a hitchhiker (alternately thumb a ride in one direction with one arm, then in the opposite direction with the other arm).

Go for a drive (using both hands, simulate turning the steering wheel of a car).

Join the army (alternately salute with one hand, then the other).

Join the circus (simulate the actions of a juggler).

Play ball.

1. First, simulate pitching the ball alternately with one arm, then the other. Gently pitch both underhand and overhand. Continue for as long as desired.

2. Then "swing the bat," taking a few swings as a right-handed batter, then a few as a left-handed batter.

Go swimming.

1. Simulate the crawl stroke. Continue for as long as desired.

2. Simulate the breast stroke. Continue for as long as desired.

3. Simulate dog-paddling.

Play a symphony.

1. Simulate playing various musical instruments that inspire energetic movements, such as the piano, trombone, violin, harp, accordion, kettle drums, and bongo drums. Continue each for as long as desired.

2. Then imitate the actions of an orchestra conductor, moving both arms about dramatically.

BASIC SEATED AEROBIC EXERCISES

As you initially get to know your participants' strengths and limitations, start your classes with the basic seated aerobic exercises. Seated exercise virtually eliminates the risk of falling.

The basic seated aerobic exercises are 10 lower-body aerobic activities (listed in table 5.3). The "Illustrated Aerobics Instruction" section at the end of this chapter illustrates and describes the 10 basic seated aerobic exercises. Teach these movements first. When your participants are ready to progress and enjoy more variety, add the corresponding upper-body movements listed as variations and progression options. To introduce additional moves and add further variety to your aerobic program, refer to the earlier section "Other Training Techniques" and the box "Developing New Aerobic Exercises."

Before leading aerobic exercises, note the following tips:

- Review the general exercise "Safety Guidelines Checklist" (in chapter 2) and "Safety Precautions for Aerobic Training" (earlier in this chapter) before leading these exercises.

- See the photographs, teaching instructions, and variations and progression options for the seated aerobic exercises at the end of this chapter.

- The seated aerobic exercises can be adapted to standing exercises.

Some elderly participants can progress to standing aerobic exercises. However, many participants in this population need to remain on a seated program, including nonambulatory participants, those with vision losses, those with balance problems that place them at high risk of falling, and frail participants at high risk of bone fractures.

BASIC STANDING AEROBIC EXERCISES

Seated lower-body aerobic exercises can be adapted to a standing position. As with the basic seated aerobic exercises, teach lower-body movements first. When your participants are ready to progress and enjoy more variety, add the corresponding upper-body movements listed as variations and progression options. To introduce additional moves and add further variety to your aerobic program, refer to the earlier section "Other Training Techniques" and the box "Developing New Aerobic Exercises."

Which participants should progress to standing aerobic exercise? Generally, those with the following characteristics:

- Can walk without assistive devices such as canes or walkers
- Can see
- Do not have balance problems that create high risk of falling
- Are not frail or at high risk of bone fractures
- Perform seated combinations of lower- and upper-body movements well

If you have any doubts, consult the participant's physician.

Standing aerobic exercises can replace seated work for qualified participants after they have become proficient with seated methods. During class, some participants can do the seated exercises while others do the standing versions. Also, a single aerobic exercise session can involve some combination of both seated and standing activity for certain individuals. For people who tolerate standing work well, the more standing aerobic exercises they perform, the better (Clark 1998).

TABLE 5.3 BASIC SEATED AEROBIC EXERCISES[a]	
Exercise	**Page**
5.1 Seated Alternate Heel Lifts	105
5.2 Seated Walking in Place	106
5.3 Seated Marching in Place	108
5.4 Seated Alternate Toe Touches to Front	109
5.5 Seated Alternate Heel Touches to Front	111
5.6 Seated Alternate Toe Touches to Sides	112
5.7 Seated Alternate Heel Touches to Sides	114
5.8 Seated Alternate Kicks	115
5.9 Seated Alternate Knee Lifts	117
5.10 Seated Alternate Double Knee Lifts	118

[a]Seated aerobic exercises can be adapted to standing exercises.

VARIATIONS AND PROGRESSION

The "Illustrated Aerobics Instruction" section at the end of the chapter gives variations and progression options for each basic seated aerobic exercise, which you may introduce after your participants have learned the basic seated exercises. As previously mentioned, including different types of aerobic exercise benefits more muscle groups, reduces the risk for overuse injury, and can improve attendance and participation rates by making your class more interesting. Create your own original exercise patterns and combinations by following the instructions provided in "Other Training Techniques," and develop new aerobic movements for your class using the ideas in "Developing New Aerobic Exercises."

Over time, gradual increases in the intensity, frequency, and duration of aerobic activity enable a participant to progress. Following are instructions for manipulating those three training variables.

As participants grow stronger, intensity can be increased very gradually within sensible limits. These are some ways to increase intensity:

- Incorporate upper-body movements along with the basic lower-body movements.
- Work at a faster speed (but always in a controlled manner).
- Work through fuller ranges of motion (lift legs higher, reach arms farther, and generally perform bigger movements).
- Progress from seated to standing activity.

When increasing the intensity for frail elderly participants, remember that RPE should never exceed 14. In this population, most progression should be achieved through slow increases in frequency and duration. Gradually, over a period of several months, frequency can be increased from three to five days per week. Likewise, duration can be increased from about 10 minutes per aerobics session to 30 minutes or longer.

Elderly participants can take up to a year to reach the maintenance stage, the stage when an individual achieves his or her desired level of health or fitness. Practically speaking, most frail elderly participants can be regarded as maintenance candidates when they can well tolerate 30-minute sessions of continuous aerobic activity at an RPE of 12 to 14, three to five days per week. At this stage, the emphasis shifts from progression to long-term, continued training (see chapter 8).

SUMMARY

Elderly fitness participants stand to gain substantially from well-designed aerobic exercise programs. Because the physical well-being of your participants is paramount, remember to err on the side of safety. By following the guidelines in this chapter, you can employ necessary safeguards without compromising the integrity of your aerobic workout or limiting your participants' fun and enthusiasm. Participants who regularly perform aerobic exercise in your class can experience major benefits, including enhanced performance, fitness, and health. In addition, the experience can be socially rewarding, both for your participants and for you!

ILLUSTRATED AEROBICS INSTRUCTION

Exercises 5.1 to 5.10 are seated and standing aerobic exercises. The "Exercise and Safety Tips" and "Variations and Progression Options" apply to both seated and standing exercises unless otherwise specified.

SEATED ALTERNATE HEEL LIFTS

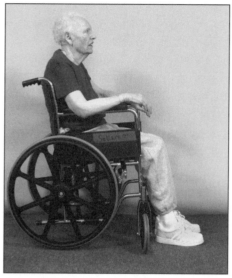

A

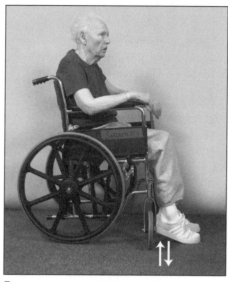

B

START/FINISH POSITION

1. Good seated posture.*
2. Hands on lap or wheelchair arms.
3. Feet flat on floor.

UPWARD/DOWNWARD MOVEMENT

4. Raise one heel off floor.
5. Lower it back onto floor.
6. Raise other heel off floor.
7. Lower it back onto floor.

Exercise and Safety Tips

- If feet are positioned too far away from chair, heel lifts will not be high enough.
- Touch heels to floor lightly to prevent bruising.
- To optimize aerobic benefits, perform heel lifts as quickly as safely possible.
- If fatigued, participants may reduce speed.
- If participants do not move in time to the musical beat during this (or any other) exercise, do not be disturbed. Simply encourage them to do their best and to enjoy themselves.
- For the standing version, pay special attention to maintaining erect posture; leaning forward compromises balance.

Variations and Progression Options

- While performing the lower-body movements, raise both arms slowly up and down while shaking fingers "Charleston-style."
- Standing Alternate Heel Lifts. Add Charleston Fingers (see photographs C and D and instructions on the next page).

(continued)

*See "Instructions for Good Seated Posture," page 63.

(continued)

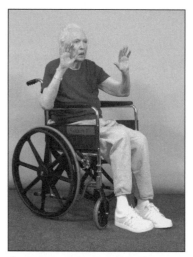

C

START/FINISH POSITION

1. Place feet flat on floor.
2. Bend elbows at sides.
3. Open hands wide.
4. Palms face front.
5. Fingers point upward.

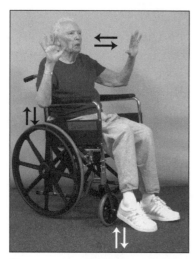

D

MOVEMENT PHASE

6. Begin Alternate Heel Lifts.
7. Shake fingers quickly from side to side.
8. Move arms slowly upward and downward.

EXERCISE 5.2	AEROBIC EXERCISE

SEATED WALKING IN PLACE

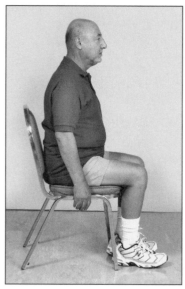

A

START/FINISH POSITION

1. Good seated posture.*
2. Arms by sides.
3. Feet flat on floor.

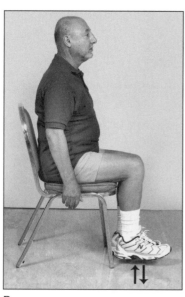

B

UPWARD/DOWNWARD MOVEMENT

4. Walk in place.

*See "Instructions for Good Seated Posture," page 63.

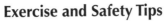

Exercise and Safety Tips

- Be sure to lower heel to floor with each step; walking on toes does not provide sufficient shock absorption.
- Touch feet to floor lightly to prevent foot injuries.
- If fatigued, seated participants may substitute Alternate Heel Lifts, and standing participants may change to the seated exercise.
- When incorporating the arm motions suggested in the "Variations and Progression Options," relax the hands and fingers to encourage circulation.
- When incorporating the suggested arm motions, swing arms energetically to optimize aerobic benefits.

Variations and Progression Options

- While walking in place, perform Alternate Arm Swings. Start with whichever arm feels more natural.
- Some participants may enjoy walking about occasionally, instead of walking in place. Walking laps (in a large circular pattern) works well indoors. Also, participants can take a certain number of steps in one direction, then in a different direction. However, note that walking backward can compromise balance.
- Standing Walking in Place. Add Alternate Arm Swings (see photographs C and D and instructions).

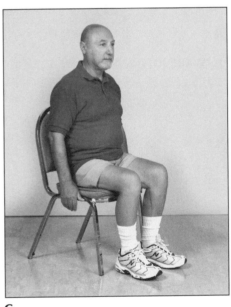

C

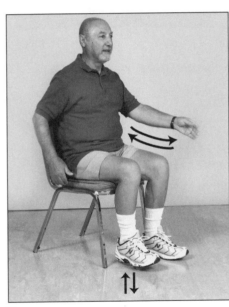

D

START/FINISH POSITION

1. Place feet flat on floor.
2. Extend both arms down at sides.
3. Relax the arms, hands, and fingers.

MOVEMENT PHASE

4. Begin Walking in Place.
5. Alternately swing one arm, then the other.
6. Swing once with each step.
7. Swing naturally, forward and backward.

SEATED MARCHING IN PLACE

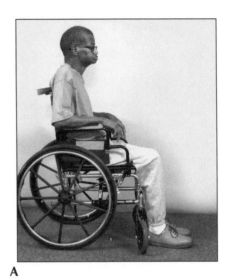

A

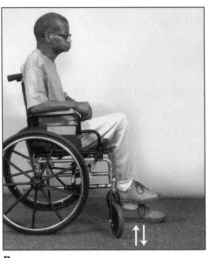

B

START/FINISH POSITION	**UPWARD/DOWNWARD MOVEMENT**
1. Good seated posture.*	4. March in place.
2. Hands on lap or wheelchair arms.	
3. Feet flat on floor.	

Exercise and Safety Tips

- Be sure to lower heel to floor with each step; marching on toes does not provide sufficient shock absorption.
- Touch feet to floor lightly to prevent foot injuries.
- If fatigued, seated participants may substitute Walking in Place, and standing participants may change to the seated exercise.
- When incorporating the arm motions suggested in "Variations and Progression Options," keep fists loose to spare the joints of the hands and fingers and to encourage circulation.
- When incorporating the suggested arm motions, swing elbows energetically to optimize aerobic benefits.

Variations and Progression Options

- While marching in place, perform Alternate Elbow Swings. Start with whichever elbow feels more natural.
- Some participants may enjoy marching about occasionally, instead of marching in place. A combination of marching and walking laps (in a large circular pattern) works well indoors. Also, participants can take a certain number of steps in one direction, then in a different direction. However, note that marching backward can compromise balance.
- Perform Standing Marching in Place. Add Alternate Elbow Swings (see photographs C and D and instructions on the next page).

*See "Instructions for Good Seated Posture," page 63.

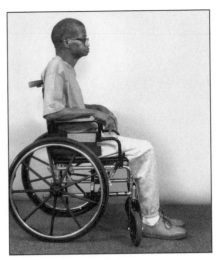

C

START/FINISH POSITION

1. Place feet flat on floor.
2. Bend elbows at sides.

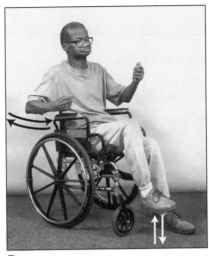

D

MOVEMENT PHASE

3. Begin Marching in Place.
4. Alternately swing one elbow, then the other.
5. Swing once with each step.
6. Swing naturally, forward and backward.

AEROBIC EXERCISE	EXERCISE 5.4

SEATED ALTERNATE TOE TOUCHES TO FRONT

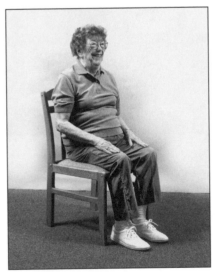

A

START/FINISH POSITION

1. Good seated posture.*
2. Hands on lap.
3. Feet flat on floor.

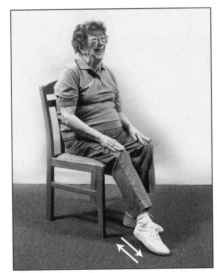

B

FORWARD/BACKWARD MOVEMENT

4. Move one foot forward, then touch toes to floor.
5. Return foot to starting position.
6. Touch toes of other foot to floor in front.
7. Return foot to starting position.

*See "Instructions for Good Seated Posture," page 63.

(continued)

(continued)

Exercise and Safety Tips

- If fatigued, seated participants may substitute Alternate Heel Lifts or Walking in Place, and standing participants may change to the seated exercise.

- When incorporating the arm motions suggested in "Variations and Progression Options," avoid slinging the arms outward. Move them in a controlled manner to protect the shoulders and elbows.

- When incorporating the suggested arm motions, people with painful arthritis in their hands should simply touch hands together rather than clapping.

- If standing, protect joints from excessive impact by keeping one foot on the floor at all times. Resist any temptation to perform a jumping version of this exercise.

Variations and Progression Options

- While performing the lower-body movements, alternately clap hands together and move arms apart.

- Standing Alternate Toe Touches to Front. Add Clapping (see photographs C and D and instructions).

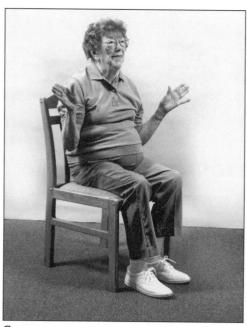

C

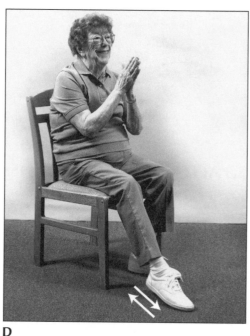

D

START/FINISH POSITION

1. Place feet flat on floor.
2. Bend elbows at sides.
3. Palms face each other.

MOVEMENT PHASE

4. Begin Alternate Toe Touches to Front.
5. Clap when toes touch front.
6. Spread arms apart when feet are together.

SEATED ALTERNATE HEEL TOUCHES TO FRONT

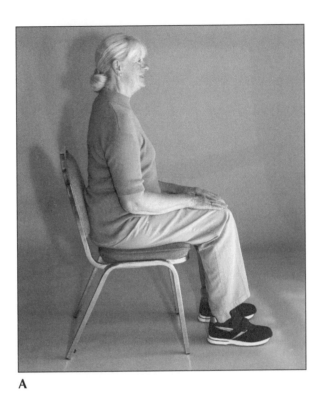

A

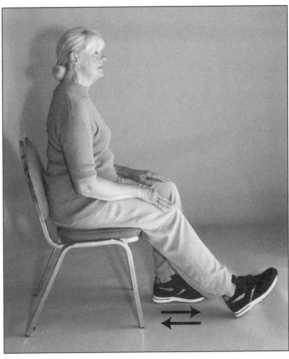

B

START/FINISH POSITION

1. Good seated posture.*
2. Hands on lap.
3. Feet flat on floor.

FORWARD/BACKWARD MOVEMENT

4. Touch one heel to floor in front.
5. Return foot to starting position.
6. Touch other heel to floor in front.
7. Return foot to starting position.

Exercise and Safety Tips

- Touch heels to floor lightly to avoid bruising.
- If fatigued, seated participants may substitute Alternate Heel Lifts or Walking in Place, and standing participants may change to the seated exercise.
- When incorporating the arm motions suggested in "Variations and Progression Options," stretch the fingers comfortably.
- If standing, protect joints from excessive impact by keeping one foot on the floor at all times. Resist any temptation to perform a jumping version of this exercise.

Variations and Progression Options

- While performing the lower-body movements, alternately reach one arm and then the other toward the front. Reach with the arm opposite the extended leg.
- Standing Alternate Heel Touches to Front. Add Alternate Reaches Toward Front (see photographs C and D and instructions on the next page).

(continued)

*See "Instructions for Good Seated Posture," page 63.

(continued)

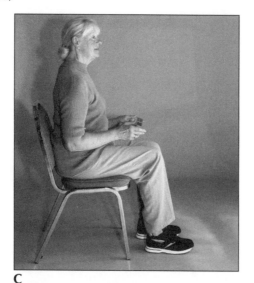

C

START/FINISH POSITION

1. Place feet flat on floor.
2. Bend elbows at sides.
3. Relax hands and fingers.

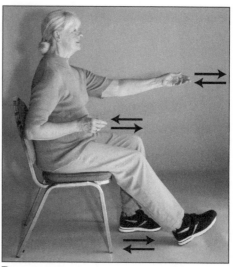

D

MOVEMENT PHASE

4. Begin Alternate Heel Touches to Front.
5. As each heel touches, reach forward with opposite arm.
6. Bend elbows at sides when feet are together.

EXERCISE 5.6	AEROBIC EXERCISE

SEATED ALTERNATE TOE TOUCHES TO SIDES

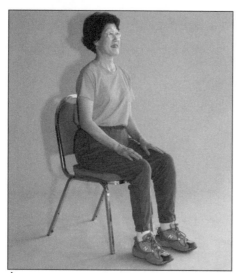

A

START/FINISH POSITION

1. Good seated posture.*
2. Hands on lap.
3. Both feet flat on floor.

*See "Instructions for Good Seated Posture," page 63.

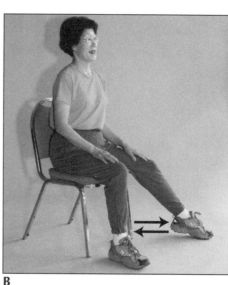

B

OUTWARD/INWARD MOVEMENT

4. Touch toes of one foot to floor at side.
5. Return foot to starting position.
6. Touch toes of other foot to floor at side.
7. Return foot to starting position.

Exercise and Safety Tips

- If fatigued, seated participants may substitute Alternate Heel Lifts, Walking in Place, or Marching in Place, and standing participants may change to the seated exercise.
- When incorporating the arm motions suggested in "Variations and Progression Options," if high arm raises are uncomfortable or impossible to perform, simply raise the arms as high as feels natural.
- If standing, protect joints from excessive impact by keeping one foot on the floor at all times. Resist any temptation to perform a jumping version of this exercise.

Variations and Progression Options

- While performing the lower-body movements, add Jumping-Jack Arms. Raise both arms high at the sides as each leg extends. Lower arms as the leg returns to starting position.
- Standing Alternate Toe Touches to Sides. Add Jumping-Jack Arms (see photographs C and D and instructions).

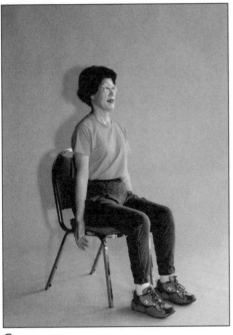

C

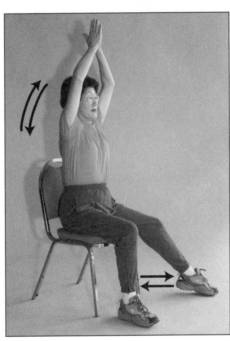

D

START/FINISH POSITION

1. Place both feet flat on floor.
2. Extend arms down at sides.

MOVEMENT PHASE

3. Begin Alternate Toe Touches to Sides.
4. As each leg extends, raise both arms.
5. Lower arms when feet are together.

SEATED ALTERNATE HEEL TOUCHES TO SIDES

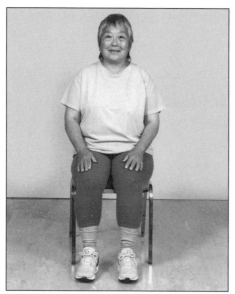

A

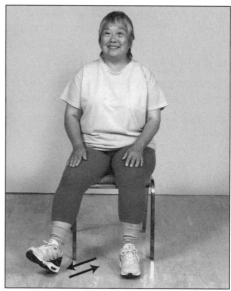

B

START/FINISH POSITION

1. Good seated posture.*
2. Hands on lap.
3. Feet flat on floor.

OUTWARD/INWARD MOVEMENT

4. Touch one heel to floor at side.
5. Return foot to starting position.
6. Touch other heel to floor at side.
7. Return foot to starting position.

Exercise and Safety Tips

- Touch heels to floor lightly to prevent bruising.
- If fatigued, seated participants may substitute Alternate Heel Lifts, Walking in Place, or Marching in Place, and standing participants may change to the seated exercise.
- If standing, protect joints from excessive impact by keeping one foot on the floor at all times. Resist any temptation to perform a jumping version of this exercise.
- When standing and extending one leg toward the side, slightly bend the opposite knee to increase range and ease of movement.
- If standing, gently turn the trunk and look to the side as each leg extends to enhance enjoyment and benefits. However, if turning causes discomfort or a light-headed feeling, keep the trunk and head facing front during limb extensions.

Variations and Progression Options

- While performing the lower-body movements, add Alternate Arm Pushes to Sides. Push both arms toward one side along with the extended leg.
- Standing Alternate Heel Touches to Sides. Add Alternate Arm Pushes to Sides (see photographs C and D and instructions on the next page).

*See "Instructions for Good Seated Posture," page 63.

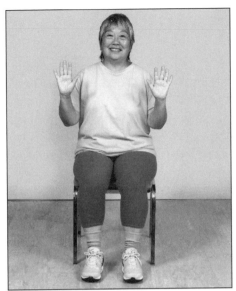

C

START/FINISH POSITION

1. Place feet flat on floor.
2. Arms in "stick 'em up" position (palms facing forward near shoulders), elbows by sides.
3. Fingers point upward.

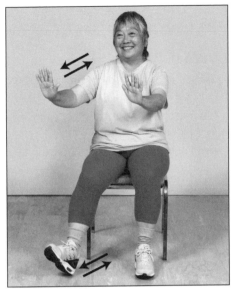

D

MOVEMENT PHASE

4. Begin Alternate Heel Touches to Sides.
5. As each leg extends, push arms along with it out to the side.
6. Bend elbows at sides when feet are together.

AEROBIC EXERCISE

SEATED ALTERNATE KICKS

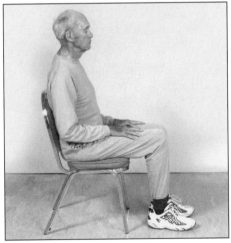

A

START/FINISH POSITION

1. Good seated posture.*
2. Hands on lap.
3. Both feet flat on floor.

*See "Instructions for Good Seated Posture," page 63.

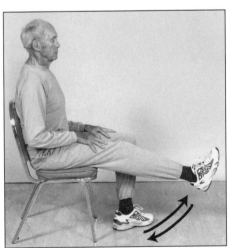

B

UPWARD/DOWNWARD MOVEMENT

4. Straighten leg.
5. Return foot to starting position.
6. Straighten other leg.
7. Return foot to starting position.

(continued)

(continued)

Exercise and Safety Tips

- If fatigued, seated participants may substitute Alternate Heel Lifts, Walking in Place, or Marching in Place, and standing participants may change to the seated exercise.
- Avoid flinging the legs during knee extensions. Move legs in a controlled manner to protect the knees (and the hips while standing).
- If standing, protect joints from excessive impact by keeping one foot on the floor at all times. Resist any temptation to perform a jumping version of this exercise.
- Although the lifted leg should be extended when standing, its knee should not be locked (rigidly straightened), which is stressful to the joint.
- If standing, lift leg to a moderate height; excessively high lifts can cause falls.

Variations and Progression Options

- While performing Alternate Kicks, swing both arms back and forth across the front.
- Standing Alternate Kicks. Add Arm Swings Across Front (see photographs C and D and instructions).

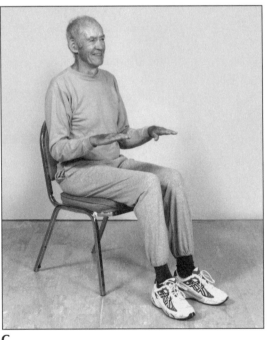

C

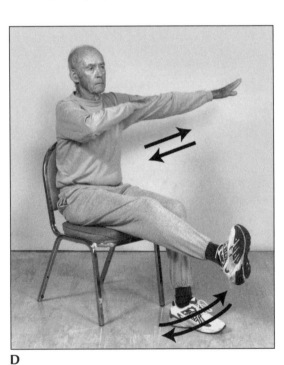

D

START/FINISH POSITION

1. Place feet flat on floor.
2. Bend elbows at sides.
3. Position hands slightly above lap.
4. Extend fingers.
5. Palms face down.

MOVEMENT PHASE

6. Begin Alternate Kicks.
7. As each leg extends, sweep arms up to opposite side.
8. Sweep arms low across lap when feet are together.

SEATED ALTERNATE KNEE LIFTS

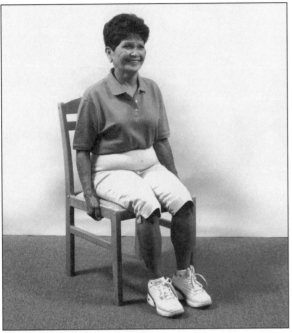

A

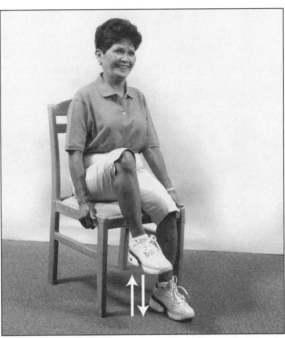

B

START/FINISH POSITION

1. Good seated posture.*
2. Hands hold side of chair.
3. Both feet flat on floor.

UPWARD/DOWNWARD MOVEMENT

4. Raise one knee high to the front.
5. Lower foot back to floor.
6. Raise other knee high to the front.
7. Lower foot back to floor.

Exercise and Safety Tips

- To prevent foot injuries, avoid stomping on the floor during this exercise.
- If fatigued, seated participants may substitute Alternate Heel Lifts, Walking in Place, or Marching in Place, and standing participants may change to the seated exercise.
- When incorporating the arm motions suggested in "Variations and Progression Options," keep fists loose during punches, never tight.
- To optimize aerobic benefits, raise knees as high as safely possible when standing, but not so high that balance is compromised.

Variations and Progression Options

- While performing Alternate Knee Lifts, perform Alternate Punches toward the front. Punch with the arm opposite the lifted knee.
- Standing Alternate Knee Lifts. Add Alternate Punches (see photographs C and D and instructions on the next page).

*See "Instructions for Good Seated Posture," page 63.

(continued)

(continued)

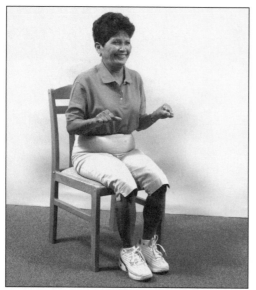

C

START/FINISH POSITION

1. Place feet flat on floor.
2. Bend elbows at sides.
3. Make loose fists.
4. Palms face down.

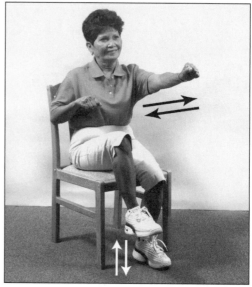

D

MOVEMENT PHASE

5. Begin Alternate Knee Lifts.
6. As each knee lifts, punch forward with opposite arm.
7. Bend elbows at sides when feet are together.

EXERCISE 5.10	AEROBIC EXERCISE

SEATED ALTERNATE DOUBLE KNEE LIFTS

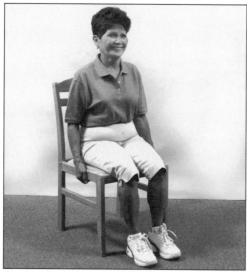

A

START/FINISH POSITION

1. Good seated posture.*
2. Hands hold side of chair.
3. Feet flat on floor.

*See "Instructions for Good Seated Posture," page 63.

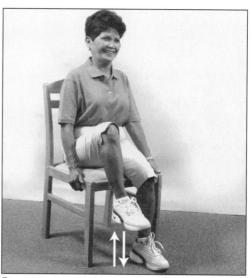

B

UPWARD/DOWNWARD MOVEMENT

4. Lift one knee high to the front.
5. Lower foot back to floor.
6. Lift same knee high to the front.

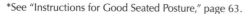

7. Lower foot back to floor.

8. Lift other knee high to the front.

9. Lower foot back to floor.

10. Lift that knee high to the front.

11. Lower foot back to floor.

Exercise and Safety Tips

- To prevent foot injuries, avoid stomping on the floor during this exercise.
- If alternate double knee lifts feel too strenuous, participants may substitute single lifts (exercise 5.9).
- When incorporating the arm motions suggested in "Variations and Progression Options," if pushing arms high overhead is uncomfortable or impossible, simply push as high as feels natural.
- To optimize aerobic benefits, lift knees as high as safely possible when standing, but not so high that balance is compromised.

Variations and Progression Options

- While performing alternate double knee lifts, perform Upward Arm Pushes.
- Standing Alternate Double Knee Lifts. Add Upward Arm Pushes (see phtographs C and D and instructions).

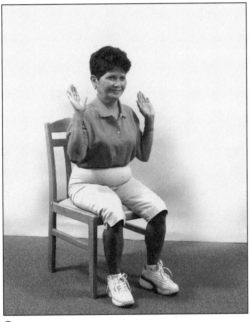

C

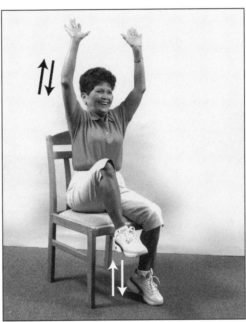

D

START/FINISH POSITION

1. Place feet flat on floor.

2. Arms in "stick 'em up" position (palms facing upward near shoulders), elbows by sides.

MOVEMENT PHASE

3. Begin Alternate Double Knee Lifts.

4. Push both arms upward with each knee lift.

CHAPTER 6

RESISTANCE TRAINING FOR MUSCULAR STRENGTH AND ENDURANCE

This chapter provides methods for teaching safe and effective resistance training (also called *strength training, progressive resistive (or resistance) training, weight training,* or *weightlifting*) for frail elders and adults with special needs. A well-rounded resistance-training program can prevent or even reverse the usual decline in strength of older adults and improve posture, balance, and functional ability. As participants increase their strength, they are better able to do daily activities requiring strength, such as getting up from a chair, climbing stairs, lifting a grandchild, and so on.

Start with the basic seated resistance exercises without weights. You will learn to safely progress to using weights and help participants who can stand to perform the basic standing resistance and balance exercises. The seated and standing exercises can be taught together, so classes can accommodate individuals at diverse levels of health and fitness. Photographs and descriptions of the resistance exercises are at the end of this chapter.

MYTHS ABOUT RESISTANCE TRAINING

Before offering resistance training to your participants, it may be helpful to debunk some common myths about weight training (table 6.1) and discuss its benefits (see appendixes A and B). This discussion can help participants be more receptive to your

class. Participants' motivation is key to program success. You may copy table 6.1, appendix A, and appendix B for easy reference and handouts.

SAFETY PRECAUTIONS FOR RESISTANCE TRAINING

Resistance training is safe for older adults if appropriate exercise guidelines and precautions are observed. The general safety precautions (page 123) and following specific safety precautions for those with special needs can help you lead safe resistance training and keep your participants injury-free. You may photocopy the "General Safety Precautions Checklist for Resistance Training" and the general exercise "Safety Guidelines Checklist" in chapter 2.

SPECIFIC SAFETY PRECAUTIONS FOR THOSE WITH SPECIAL NEEDS

Following are some specific safety precautions for leading resistance exercises for people with specific needs. These may not apply to every individual with a particular condition. For example, an individual with mild symptoms of arthritis may have few limitations on resistance exercises, whereas severe symptoms may prohibit resistance training. Also, remember that an individual's performance

TABLE 6.1   COMMON MYTHS AND FACTS ABOUT RESISTANCE TRAINING

Myth	Fact
"You have to be in shape first."	Generally, the more out of shape you are, the more you can benefit from resistance training.
"I don't need resistance training because I do aerobics."	Aerobic exercise is great for cardiovascular fitness, but resistance training for muscular strength and endurance rounds out an exercise program.
"Weight training is for men."	Women of all ages as well as men can significantly benefit from resistance training programs.
"I don't want to develop large, bulky muscles." (women)	Most women's genetic makeup prevents them from developing the large muscles that men can acquire when using weights.
"Weight training requires heavy barbells and other special equipment."	Lighter and less expensive weights can work just as effectively as heavy barbells and other special equipment.
"No pain, no gain."	"Train, don't strain" or "No pain, you gain" is a more sensible approach to resistance training.
"Weight training is hard on the joints."	Sensible resistance exercise can improve joint strength.
"It takes too much time."	All you need is one set of 8 to 12 repetitions of 8 to 10 exercises that condition the major muscle groups, at least twice a week.
"It won't help me lose excess fat weight."	An increase in muscle mass increases your metabolism, which makes it easier to lose fat weight.
"When you quit resistance training, your muscle turns to fat."	The result of detraining is muscle loss. If you keep eating as much as you were during training but don't burn it off with exercise, you will gain fat.
"It takes more willpower and discipline than I have."	One of the many benefits you can gain from resistance training is more energy for daily activities.
"I'm too old to lift weights."	People in their 90s, including nursing home residents, can weight-train safely and increase muscle strength significantly.

From *Exercise for Frail Elders* by E. Best-Martini and K. A. Botenhagen-DiGenova, 2003, Champaign, IL: Human Kinetics.

ability can vary from day to day. See chapter 1 to learn more about common medical disorders in the elderly. Above all, follow the physician's or physical therapist's special exercise recommendations for the participant.

ALZHEIMER'S DISEASE AND RELATED DEMENTIAS

- Do not use rigid *free weights* (handheld weights, such as dumbbells or canned foods), which can cause injury if dropped. A safer alternative is wrist weights or an improvised weight such as a 1-pound bag of beans in a sock.

- Since confused or disoriented participants may be unable to rate perceived exertion dependably, be especially vigilant of their response to resistance training.

ARTHRITIS

- Short, frequent exercise sessions are better tolerated than long, less frequent ones. For example, instead of combining resistance training and aerobics into a 1-hour class on Mondays, Wednesdays, and Fridays, people with arthritis might respond more favorably to 30 minutes of resistance exercise on Mondays and Fridays and 30 minutes of aerobic activity on Tuesdays, Thursdays, and Saturdays. Two days of resistance training per week are generally better tolerated than three days per week.

- Gradually build up to 10 to 12 repetitions with light resistance (RPE of 10 to 11; see figure 5.1, page 99).

- Mild isometric exercises can strengthen the joint and surrounding muscles without harm.

General Safety Precautions Checklist for Resistance Training

❏ Review the physician's or physical therapist's special recommendations or comments for a participant on the "Statement of Medical Clearance for Exercise" (appendix C).

❏ Remind participants to observe recommendations from their physician or physical therapist.

❏ Always warm up for at least 10 minutes before and cool down for at least 10 minutes after resistance training.

❏ Demonstrate all weight-training exercises in a slow, controlled manner.

❏ Avoid jerking or thrusting weights into position. This can cause injuries.

❏ Instruct your participants never to hold their breath while lifting, as it increases chest pressure, which may restrict blood return to the heart and markedly elevate blood pressure. Also, breath holding can increase intraabdominal pressure and cause a hernia.

❏ In general, avoid *isometric resistance* (muscles' contracting against resistance in a stationary position with no joint movement) exercises that can raise blood pressure.

❏ Do not grip hand weights too tightly. Use a relaxed grip.

❏ Keep wrists in a *neutral position* (straight) during all upper-body resistance exercises.

❏ Lift arms and legs only as high as comfortable while maintaining erect posture.

❏ Avoid hyperextending or locking the joints. When standing, avoid locking the knee of the supporting leg; keep the knee soft, not bent.

❏ While performing the lower-body resistance exercises, always keep one foot on the floor at all times.

❏ If participants experience pain in or near a joint when using weights, have them stop the exercise. See figure 2.1 in chapter 2 for further information.

❏ Do not overtrain. Mild muscle soreness lasting up to a few days and slight fatigue are normal after resistance training, but exhaustion, sore joints, and unpleasant muscle soreness are not.

❏ Use the same amount of weight on each side for the upper- and lower-body resistance exercises.

❏ Remove leg weights before walking around. Walking with leg weights can increase risk of falling.

❏ When the weights are not being used, place them in a safe place, perhaps under participants' chairs, so no one will trip over them.

❏ Prevent participants' falling forward and a possible increase in cranial pressure by instructing them not to lower their heads below parallel with the floor when bending forward, as when picking up or putting down weights.

From *Exercise for Frail Elders* by E. Best-Martini and K. A. Botenhagen-DiGenova, 2003, Champaign, IL: Human Kinetics.

INSTRUCTIONS FOR ISOMETRIC EXERCISES

- We recommended isometrics *only* when working one-on-one with participants without hypertension. Make sure they continuously breathe while holding weights, because breath holding and isometric exercise both increase blood pressure. The "Instructions for Isometric Exercises" are aimed at increasing muscle strength without significantly increasing blood pressure.

- Do not permit participants with arthritis to do isotonic resistance exercises with weights during acute phases of pain or inflammation. They can perform the resistance exercises without weights.

- Start with one isometric contraction per exercise; slowly progress to six if well tolerated. Initially hold contractions for 3 seconds per contraction; slowly progress to 6 seconds, if well tolerated. Rest for 20 seconds between contractions. The contraction can be held at different points throughout the pain-free range of motion of a resistance exercise. An isometric contraction performed at one joint angle strengthens the muscle only at that specific angle. For this reason, repetitions at different joint angles are beneficial.

- During rest periods, practice a breathing, range of motion (see chapter 4), or stretching exercise (particularly one for the muscle that is being contracted; see chapter 7). When acute pain, swelling, and inflammation go away, or at least subside, see how the participant responds to *isotonic resistance exercises* (exercises involving contractions against resistance with joint movement, i.e., typical free-weight training) through the full pain-free range of motion of an exercise.

- Ask participants how they felt after the previous resistance class, and make appropriate modifications in the next session to prevent overtraining.

CHRONIC OBSTRUCTIVE PULMONARY DISEASE

- It is especially important to prevent straining the respiratory and cardiovascular systems. For example, avoid sustained isometrics, holding the breath, heavy weight training (at an RPE of 15, "Hard (heavy)" or more), and holding any weight overhead for more than a few seconds.

CORONARY ARTERY DISEASE (HEART DISEASE)

- "Mild-to-moderate resistance training can provide a safe and effective method for improving muscular strength and endurance in selected cardiac individuals" (American College of Sports Medicine 1997, 25). A participant's physician should indicate whether or not resistance training is recommended.

- Cardiac patients should not resistance-train if they have any of the following conditions: uncontrolled hypertension, symptomatic congestive heart failure, uncontrolled arrhythmias, severe valvular disease, or unstable symptoms.

- The American College of Sports Medicine (1994, 3) recommends starting with 10 to 12 repetitions with weights that can be lifted comfortably. Increase weight when 12 to 15 repetitions can be completed comfortably.

- Avoid straining by using the RPE scale (see figure 5.1 in chapter 5). The American Association of Cardiovascular and Pulmonary Rehabilitation (1999, 113) recommends an RPE ranging from "light" (11) to "somewhat hard" (13). Have participants check with their physicians before increasing the resistance higher than 11.

- Avoid actions that excessively raise blood pressure (see the special precautions for COPD and hypertension).

- Stop exercising at the first signs or symptoms of overexertion or cardiac complications, particularly dizziness, abnormal heart rhythm, unusual shortness of breath, or chest discomfort. Refer to the section "Emergencies" in chapter 2 for guidelines about when to seek immediate medical attention. Remind participants to let you know if they have any discomfort or cardiac symptoms.

DIABETES

- Light weight training (RPE of 10 to 11) is recommended when blood pressure is normal, unless otherwise indicated by the participant's physician.

DEPRESSION

- Lifting heavier weights may be more effective for reducing depression. We recommend using heavier weight (more than 8 pounds, or 3.6 kilograms) only with medical clearance for the use of heavier weights, when working with the participant one-on-one or in a small class, and if it does not compromise the participant's enjoyment.

- If safe and appropriate for the participant, slightly increase the resistance when 11 repetitions (rather than 12 to 15) are completed with good technique in at least two consecutive workouts. If the response to this increase is positive, consider increasing the resistance again when participant can complete 10 repetitions in at least two successive sessions. Never do fewer than eight repetitions of a resistance exercise.

FRAILTY

- Begin frail elders with about four resistance exercises performed at a low intensity (start with no weight, then 0.5 pound, or 0.2 kilogram). As their strength increases, encourage them to do more exercises and gradually lift more weight.

- Ankle and wrist weights are handy for frail elderly.

- Resistance-train three times per week.

HIP FRACTURE OR REPLACEMENT

- Most patients are ready to start resistance training six months after hip surgery.

- They may need to work with their physical therapist to modify the resistance exercises.

- Avoid resistance exercises that involve internal rotation (turning the leg inward), hip adduction (crossing the legs), and hip flexion of more than 90 degrees (thigh higher than parallel with the floor) to prevent the risk of hip dislocation. Participants in chairs that allow their knees to be lower than their hips and who are able to follow directions can be asked to raise their feet (one at a time) 1 inch (2.5 centimeters) off the floor or less for the Seated Hip Flexion (exercise 6.7). During Modified Chair Stands and Chair Stands (exercise 6.6), instruct participants to keep their torsos as erect as possible (to lean forward as little as possible). For the Standing Hip Abduction and Adduction (exercise 6.8), bring the leg only to the midline of the body (do not cross one leg in front of the other).

HYPERTENSION

- Avoid any exercises that can excessively raise blood pressure, such as heavy weight lifting (at an RPE of 15 "Hard (heavy)" or more), sustained isometric muscular contractions, excessive overhead arm exercise, gripping the exercise accessories or equipment too hard, strong-grip exercises using hard rubber balls, and holding the breath.

- Use a light weight (RPE of 10 to 11) and more repetitions (12 to 15), unless otherwise recommended by participant's physician.

MULTIPLE SCLEROSIS AND PARKINSON'S DISEASE

- Have participants with Parkinson's disease and Multiple Sclerosis use light weights (0.5–3 pounds, or 0.2–1.4 kilograms), if safe and well tolerated.

- For some individuals, such as those with mild symptoms, heavier weights may be beneficial.

- Alternate between resistance and aerobic training in successive classes.

OSTEOPOROSIS

- With the physician approval, start with light forms of resistance, such as low-tension exercise bands, soft putty, sponges, or Nerf® balls.

- Gradually progress to light (0.5 pound, or 0.2 kilogram) handheld or wrist weights. If symptoms such as pain or reduced function arise from light handheld weights, go back to lighter forms of resistance.

- When osteoporosis is advanced, standing exercise may not be safe because of the risk of falling and because body weight alone can fracture spinal vertebrae. Stay with the seated exercises to eliminate the risk of falling.

- Avoid resistance exercises that involve spinal flexion, particularly in combination with stooping, which increases the risk of vertebral fractures. During the Chair Stand (exercise 6.6), maintain the natural curves of the spine by moving the head, neck, and spine as one unit throughout the exercise.

- A helpful visualization to ensure good posture is to have participants imagine a string attached to the top of the head, pulling gently upward as they sit and stand.

SENSORY LOSSES

- Use visual cues as often as possible, such as demonstration of the resistance exercises, for participants with hearing loss.
- Describe resistance exercises precisely and directly to participants with visual impairment.

GUIDELINES FOR RESISTANCE TRAINING

Several prominent organizations have developed guidelines for safe and effective resistance training, including the American College of Sports Medicine (1998a, 1998b), the American Council on Exercise (Cotton et al. 1998), the American Senior Fitness Association (2003b), the National Strength and Conditioning Association (Earle and Baechle 2000), and the YMCA of the USA (1994, 2000). Table 6.2 is a synthesis of their resistance-training guidelines for older adults. The resistance exercises in this chapter are based on these well-researched guidelines. You may make a copy of table 6.2 for easy reference and as an educational handout for your participants.

The following sections present more detailed information about the guidelines to minimize injury and maximize the benefits of resistance training for frail elders and adults with special needs.

EXERCISE SELECTION

Resistance training classes should include an initial warm-up period (see chapter 4), a minimum of eight resistance exercises, and a final cool-down period (see chapter 7). This chapter provides five upper-body and seven lower-body basic resistance

TABLE 6.2	GENERAL RESISTANCE-TRAINING GUIDELINES FOR OLDER ADULTS
Exercise selection	At least eight safe exercises that condition the major muscle groups of the body.
Exercise sequence	During light resistance training, move from head to toe or from toe to head. During light or intensive resistance training, move from larger to smaller muscle groups, postural muscles last.
Intensity (amount of weight or resistance)	Initially, perform 8 to 15 repetitions at an exertion level perceived as very light to light (an RPE of 9 to 11). Progress to "somewhat hard" (an RPE of 12 to 14) when appropriate, after excellent technique is learned.
Frequency	Two to three times per week on nonconsecutive days when doing a full-body workout.
Number of repetitions	Eight to 15 repetitions in a row per set. Begin with eight repetitions.
Range of motion	Exercise through the full, pain-free range of joint movement without hyperextending.
Speed	Slow, smooth movement. Take 3 seconds to lift or push a weight into place, and take another 3 seconds to return the weight to the start/finish position.
Number of sets	One to three sets per exercise.
Rest periods between sets	Wait at least 1 to 2 minutes between sets of 8 to 15 repetitions.
Rest periods between exercises	The rest period can be longer (up to 1 minute) if heavier resistance is used, and can be shortened or eliminated with lighter resistance, as the individual's tolerance to exercise increases over time.
Rest periods between workouts	At least 48 hours of rest between full-body workouts.
Progression and maintenance	Gradually increase resistance by increments of 1 pound (0.5 kilogram) or less. Reduce repetitions to 8; progress gradually to 12 to 15 repetitions at the heavier weight. Alternatively, add a second set of 8 repetitions, and gradually progress to 15. When participants reach long-term resistance training goals, encourage lifetime maintenance.

From *Exercise for Frail Elders* by E. Best-Martini and K. A. Botenhagen-DiGenova, 2003, Champaign, IL: Human Kinetics.

exercises that condition the major muscle groups of the body (identified in tables 6.3 and 6.5), with the exception of the abdominal (postural) muscles that cannot be safely exercised with resistance while sitting. Participants can strengthen the postural muscles by performing resistance exercises sitting *upright* (not leaning against the back of the chair). Teach the basic seated resistance exercises first. Participants who are stable on their feet can progress to standing resistance and balance exercises.

EXERCISE SEQUENCE

Follow the given order of the exercises, which goes from larger to smaller muscle groups. This is the order recommended for intensive resistance training, but it is appropriate for both light and intensive resistance training.

TRAINING INTENSITY

Initially, teach the resistance exercises without weights. Participants will be encouraged to learn that lifting the weight of their arms and legs alone is beneficial. When they have learned the exercises, begin with light weights, such as 1 pound (0.5 kilogram). In the section "Basic Seated Resistance Exercises" later in this chapter, you will learn how to teach the exercises without weights and the essentials of introducing weights.

How much weight an individual lifts depends on his or her medical status, exercise tolerance, and goals. When starting with weights, perform 8 to 15 repetitions at an exertion level perceived as very light to light (an RPE of 9 to 11). You can use the RPE scale (see figure 5.1 in chapter 5) to help participants find an appropriate training intensity. After participants learn excellent technique, gradually progress to 12 or 14 ("somewhat hard") on the RPE scale, when appropriate. "Somewhat hard" should not involve any strain or pain. We recommend avoiding terms such as *fatigue* or *muscular failure,* which can have negative connotations.

TRAINING FREQUENCY

We recommend that you initially schedule resistance training two days per week on nonconsecutive days. After your participants respond favorably to resistance training for several months, try three times per week. This increases the chance that your participants can make it to class at least a minimum of two times per week. Especially encourage frail elders and others with sedentary lifestyles to attend class three times per week. Encourage beginners to your class to start with two days and gradually progress to three.

NUMBER OF REPETITIONS

Begin teaching 8 to 10 repetitions per *set* (a separate bout of an exercise) of each resistance exercise. Work up to 12 to 15 repetitions per set. Doing 15 repetitions makes it easier to progress to a heavier weight. When a participant reaches 12 to 15 repetitions, it is time to increase the weight and decrease the repetitions back to 8. If some participants are doing fewer repetitions than others, they must wait for the others to complete the extra repetitions. Therefore, with a class, we suggest a maximum of 12 repetitions to minimize the waiting time of those doing fewer repetitions.

TRAINING RANGE OF MOTION

Earle and Baechle (2000, 345) stated, "When the entire range of motion (ROM) is covered during an exercise, the value of the exercise is maximized and flexibility is maintained or improved." Remind your participants to lift weights through their full, pain-free range of motion (the maximum range of joint movement that does not elicit discomfort or pain) without hyperextending or locking their joints. They should feel the exercises in their muscles and not in their joints.

TRAINING SPEED

Take 3 to 4 seconds to lift or push a weight into place, and take another 3 to 4 seconds to lower the weight while resisting gravity. The count for resistance training is slow, (e.g., "1, 1, 1, up, 1, 1, 1, down; 2, 2, 2, up, ...)" Refer to the discussion of counting in the section "Step 1: Demonstrate and Describe" and table 3.3 in chapter 3. Have participants count aloud while learning resistance exercise to reinforce slow movement.

NUMBER OF SETS

One to three sets of 8 to 15 repetitions per exercise is a general recommendation for strength training. Start with one set. Remember that it is better to do one set slowly with good technique than to do two or three sets quickly. (There is not strong evidence that more than one set produces greater strength gains.)

REST PERIODS BETWEEN SETS, EXERCISES, AND WORKOUTS

Wait 1 to 2 minutes before doing a second or third set of 8 to 15 repetitions. Between sets, try two-part deep-breathing (chapter 4), range-of-motion exercises (chapter 4), or stretching exercises (chapter 7).

In general, give longer rest periods between exercises with heavier resistance. Shorten or eliminate rest periods between different exercises of lighter resistance, as participants' tolerance to exercise improves. Finally, schedule resistance training so that your participants have at least 48 hours of rest between full-body workouts.

PROGRESSION AND MAINTENANCE

When participants can easily complete 12 to 15 repetitions of a resistance exercise, they may progress in either of these ways:

1. Slightly increase the amount of weight (ideally, by 1 pound [0.5 kilogram] or less) and drop back to eight repetitions. With resistance bands or tubes, increase to a firmer band of slightly more resistance. Gradually progress to a maximum of 12 to 15 repetitions at the heavier resistance.

2. Add a second set of initially 8 repetitions, and gradually progress to 15. Less weight can be used for the second set.

See chapter 8 for more information about progression.

Work with participants' physicians and physical therapists to set weight-training goals. We recommend using dumbbells weighing between 1 and 10 pounds (0.5 and 4.5 kilograms) and that participants increase their weights in 1-pound (0.5-kilogram) increments. In helping participants set realistic resistance weight goals, bear in mind that frail elders and many adults with special needs are generally not able to exercise with 10-pound (4.5-kilogram) or heavier weights. A safe goal for people with dementia or advanced osteoporosis may be using 1-pound weights for both the upper- and lower-body exercises. On the other hand, someone with a hip replacement might not be able to use any additional weight for lower-body resistance exercises but may eventually reach 10 pounds for the upper-body exercises. In general, with this population it is not safe or feasible to use weights heavier than 10 pounds (4.5 kilograms).

Some participants cannot realize their resistance-training goals in a class setting. In such cases, if it is appropriate, recommend that they join a local fitness facility or hire a qualified personal trainer.

When it is appropriate for a participant to cease progressing and begin maintaining his or her current level of resistance training depends on his or her goals, motivation, physical and mental ability, physician's or physical therapist's recommenda-

tions, and available equipment. See chapter 8 for more information about maintenance.

A key to success in resistance training is recording participants' attendance and progress. The Resistance Training Log in appendix K, which you may copy, enables you and your participants to track weight and repetitions of each resistance exercise. At least once per month, make time at the beginning or end of class to evaluate the resistance training log with each participant. In the meantime, encourage participants to let you know how they are doing so that you can make appropriate adjustments. See chapter 8 for more information about monitoring attendance and progress.

OTHER TRAINING TECHNIQUES

- Maintain good seated or standing posture when performing resistance exercises.

- Before performing each exercise, instruct participants to stabilize their shoulders by moving them up, back, and down and to keep their shoulders down throughout each exercise.

- Instruct participants to "focus on" or "feel" the major muscles that are being exercised.

- Breathe continuously throughout every repetition. Prevent breath holding by one of these methods:

  1. Count aloud with each repetition (particularly with beginners and larger classes). Participants cannot hold their breath if they are speaking.

  2. Have participants practice *optimal breathing* after they learn to lift the weight slowly and safely while counting. For optimal breathing, breathe out as you lift or push the weight, and breathe in as you return the weight to the starting position. This breathing pattern feels natural after it is practiced for a while.

- You may insert a ROM exercise between resistance exercises. Pick an exercise that loosens up the body part just worked. For example, after a Chest Press (exercise 6.1), which works the chest and shoulders, try a Shoulder Rotation (exercise 4.15), which loosens up the chest and shoulders.

- Stretch each muscle group after strength training. See the stretching exercises in chapter 7.

- Anyone returning to resistance training after a significant time off should start at half his or her usual training intensity, then gradually increase the resistance.

BASIC SEATED RESISTANCE EXERCISES

The basic seated resistance exercises include five upper-body exercises and seven lower-body exercises. Familiarize yourself with the functional role of each resistance exercise, given in table 6.3. It is inspiring for your participants to hear how an exercise helps them perform daily activities. Also, learn—and teach to your participants—the body parts and major muscles (also called *prime mover muscles*, the muscles primarily responsible for performing a spe-

cific movement) targeted by each resistance exercise (see appendix J). This knowledge can help your participants focus on the body part or muscles they are strengthening. You may make a copy of appendix J and table 6.3 to refer to during class.

Before leading the seated resistance exercises, note the following tips:

- Review the general exercise "Safety Guidelines Checklist" (in chapter 2) and the section "Safety Precautions for Resistance Training" (earlier in this chapter) before leading these exercises.

TABLE 6.3 BASIC SEATED RESISTANCE EXERCISES

Target body parts and major muscles	Seated upper-body resistance exercises	Functional role[a]	Page
Chest (pectoralis major) Back of upper arms (triceps) Shoulders (deltoids)	*6.1 Seated Chest Press	Pushing a door open, pushing up from a lying position	135
Back (latissimus dorsi, trapezius) Front of upper arms (biceps) Shoulders (deltoids)	*6.2 Seated Two-Arm Row	Pulling a door open, posture	136
Shoulders (deltoids) Back of upper arms (triceps)	*6.3 Seated Overhead Press	Lifting (especially overhead)	138
Front of upper arms (biceps)	6.4 Seated Biceps Curl	Lifting, pulling	139
Back of upper arms (triceps)	6.5 Seated Triceps Extension (challenger)	Pushing, pressing up from seated or lying position	140
Target body parts and major muscles	**Seated lower-body resistance exercises**	**Functional role[a]**	**Page**
Thighs (quadriceps, hamstrings) Buttocks (gluteals)	*6.6 Modified Chair Stands (challenger)	Stand from sitting, stair climbing, walking (forward progression and stability)	141
Front hips and thighs (hip flexors)	*6.7 Seated Hip Flexion	Stair climbing, pelvic tilt, posture	143
Outer hips and thighs (hip abductors) Inner thighs (hip adductors)	*6.8 Seated Hip Abduction and Adduction	Hip rotation (lateral or medial), pelvic stabilization, posture, walking	144
Back of thighs (hamstrings)	6.9 Seated Knee Flexion	Walking (foot clearance)	146
Front of thighs (quadriceps)	6.10 Seated Knee Extension	Stand from sitting, stair climbing, walking (forward progression and stability)	147
Shins (tibialis anterior)	*6.11 Seated Toe Raises	Walking (foot clearance)	149
Calves (gastrocnemius, soleus)	*6.12 Seated Heel Raises	Walking (push-off)	150

[a]Adapted, by permission, from S. McKelvey, 2003, *Functional fitness for older adults training manual* (San Diego, CA: Aging and Independent Services), 7.

*The eight exercises preceded by an asterisk are recommended for a shorter program.

From *Exercise for Frail Elders* by E. Best-Martini and K. A. Botenhagen-DiGenova, 2003, Champaign, IL: Human Kinetics.

- See the photographs, teaching instructions, and variations and progression options at the end of this chapter.

- Seated upper- and lower-body resistance exercises can be adapted to standing exercises. See the section "Basic Standing Resistance and Balance Exercises" later in this chapter.

- The eight exercises marked by an asterisk in table 6.3 are recommended for a shorter program.

- Introduce the two challenger exercises (6.5. Seated Triceps Extension and 6.6 Modified Chair Stands) after participants have learned the other basic exercises.

Before teaching the resistance exercises, be sure to review the guidelines and safety precautions for resistance training. If you are a beginner fitness leader or would like to enhance your leadership skills, review the three-step instructional process (chapter 3). Teach the basic seated resistance exercises before the standing resistance exercises. Participants who are able to stand safely can slowly progress to the standing resistance exercises. The Modified Chair Stand is included with the seated exercises as a means of progression from the sitting to the standing exercises. Participants who are at risk of falling should have an assistant by their side for this exercise.

START WITHOUT WEIGHTS

Many older adults may require an initial training period to get into shape before lifting a weight. For instance, beginners with a low level of fitness can perform the arm and leg movements without resistance equipment. This technique is called *body-weight exercise*. The weight of the arms and legs provides sufficient resistance while doing the exercises without weights, particularly for those who have led sedentary lifestyles.

Despite a particular individual's initial level of fitness, begin teaching resistance training exercises without weights. Begin with a few exercises, for instance, just lower-body exercises, for the first week or so. Introduce upper-body exercises after the participants are comfortable with the lower-body exercises. Begin with one set of eight repetitions of each exercise, if possible. Defer introducing free weights until your participants can perform 12 repetitions without weights with good technique.

INTRODUCING WEIGHTS

After learning the basic seated resistance exercises without weights, your participants can start using weights that are 1 pound (0.5 kilogram) or lighter. How do you know when participants are ready to use weights?

- They have learned good exercise technique using just their body weight.

- They can comfortably do 12 repetitions of each exercise.

Reassure participants who are unable to perform 12 repetitions using just their body weight for resistance that they will slowly but surely get stronger. Participants with a higher initial level of fitness can start using weights sooner. "Some individuals may progress to a heavier weight in a few days, whereas others may take weeks or may never progress beyond a small weight" (Brown-Watson 1999, 101). A participant who is using a *resistive device* (all forms of resistance other than just body weight) should be able to do at least eight repetitions of each exercise. If not, decrease the resistance until the participant can do at least eight repetitions.

UPPER-BODY WEIGHTS

Each participant in your fitness class who is ready to use weights should have access to a minimum of two pairs of upper-body weights: a moderate weight and a heavier weight. Table 6.4 can help you pick two weights for each person. Start with just the moderate weight, 1 pound (0.5 kilogram) or less. Progress to a moderate and heavier pair of 1 and 2 (.9 kilogram) pounds when a participant is ready. Avoid large discrepancies in weight lifted by *opposing muscle groups* (muscles that produce the opposite joint movement), such as chest and back, or biceps and triceps.

Bear in mind that you may need to adjust the general weight recommendations in table 6.4 for individual participants. Day-to-day variations in weight-lifting ability are common. For instance, if a participant suffered from insomnia the night before class, he or she may not be able to lift as much as usual. Additionally, if your class is large, if you do not have assistance, or if it would be unsafe for participants to reach down to switch weights, participants should use only one pair of weights for all the upper-body exercises or use resistance bands or tubes. Participants who use bands or tubes should start with a band of light resistance for all upper-body resistance exercises. Then progress to using two bands—*separately for specific exercises*—one band of light resistance for exercises requiring a "moderate" weight and another of the next higher resis-

TABLE 6.4 GUIDELINES FOR CHOOSING UPPER-BODY WEIGHTS

Each row of moderate and heavier weights represents an appropriate weight range. For example, if a 3-pound weight can be used for an exercise that calls for moderate weight, use 5 pounds for heavier-weight exercises.

Moderate weights	Heavier weights	Use moderate weight with these exercises	Use heavier weight with these exercises
1 pound (0.5 kilogram)	2 pounds (0.9 kilogram)	• Chest Press[b]	• Overhead Press
2 pounds (0.9 kilogram)	3 pounds (1.4 kilograms)	• Two-Arm Row[b]	• Biceps Curl
3 pounds (1.4 kilograms)	5 pounds (2.3 kilograms)	• Triceps Extension	• Chair Stands[c]
4 pounds[a] (1.8 kilograms)	6 pounds[a] (2.7 kilograms)		
5 pounds (2.3 kilograms)	7 or 8 pounds[a] (3.2 or 3.6 kilograms)		
6 pounds[a] (2.7 kilograms)	9 pounds[a] (4.1 kilograms)		
7 pounds[a] (3.2 kilograms)	10 pounds (4.5 kilograms)		
8 pounds (3.6 kilograms)	10 or 12 pounds (4.5 or 5.4 kilograms)		

Adapted, by permission, from S. McKelvey, 2003, *Functional fitness for older adults training manual* (San Diego, CA: Aging and Independent Services), 17-18.

[a]If you use cast-iron weights in your class, ignore the 4-, 6-, 7-, and 9-pound weight options; these weights are not available in cast iron.

[b]Performing the Chest Press and Two-Arm Row in an upright, seated position puts greater demand on the smaller shoulder muscles if weights are used. Therefore, we recommend using a moderate weight for these exercises. When using resistance bands, which are not influenced by gravity or body position, bands of greater resistance can be used for these exercises.

[c]Chair Stands, a lower-body exercise, can be done with hand weights when participants are ready to make the exercise more challenging.

tance for exercises requiring a "heavier" weight (see table 6.4).

Consider safety and the special needs of your participants when selecting exercise equipment for resistance training. For example, participants who have problems holding on to a dumbbell can use wrist weights or weights with handles. Resistance bands and tubes can be a good choice for participants who cannot safely handle weights. They can also be more effective than free weights for certain seated upper-body resistance exercises, such as the Seated Chest Press and Seated Two-Arm Row. For more information on resistance bands and tubes, see the "Suggested Resources."

LOWER-BODY WEIGHTS

Use the same weight for all the lower-body exercises. It is time-consuming and unnecessary to vary the amount of weight in a class with individuals who require assistance. Leg weights can be more expensive than hand weights, so it is common for participants to make do with one weight by switching it from one leg to the other. Participants who are unable to switch a single leg weight from leg to leg need weights for both legs, unless you or an assistant can help with attaching and removing the weights. For classes with consistent members, it is ideal to label leg weights with participants' names. This is an easy way to keep track of the weight lifted by each individual.

BASIC STANDING RESISTANCE AND BALANCE EXERCISES

The basic standing resistance and balance exercises include five upper-body and seven lower-body exercises (see table 6.5). These exercises can replace the basic seated resistance exercises after your participants have become proficient at them. Some participants can do the seated exercises while others do standing exercises. We recommend that participants with major balance problems continue to do the seated lower-body resistance exercises unless they have medical clearance for standing exercises and an experienced assistant to help them with each exercise. A participant who has balance problems should perform only those standing exercises that leave a hand available to hold on to a stable support. Only those who are steady on their feet should perform the standing upper-body exercises that require weights or bands in both hands. You may make a copy of table 6.5 to refer to during class.

Before leading the standing resistance and balance exercises, note the following tips:

- Start with the basic seated resistance exercises.
- The standing resistance and balance exercises are given as variations and progression options for the basic seated resistance exercises in the section "Illustrated Resistance-Training Instruction" at the end of this chapter.
- If a participant has difficulty with a standing exercise, he or she can do the corresponding seated exercise.
- The eight exercises marked by an asterisk in table 6.5 are recommended for a shorter program.
- Introduce the two challenger exercises (6.5. Standing Triceps Extension and 6.6 Chair Stands) after participants have learned the other exercises.

STANDING UPPER-BODY RESISTANCE EXERCISES

The seated upper-body resistance exercises can be adapted to a standing position. In general, however, we recommend that the upper-body resistance exercises be performed seated, especially exercises that require weights in both hands. Exercising with weights is generally safer in a seated position, which makes it easier to concentrate on the working muscles. The standing lower-body resistance and balance exercises keep both hands free to hold on to a support (such as a steady chair) and can improve balance.

If you are working one-on-one with someone who does not have major balance problems, you may want to vary his or her weight-training regimen by doing some or all of the upper-body exercises standing. If your client has minor balance problems, have a chair close enough that it will be easy to help your client sit down if he or she loses his or her balance. Refer to the variations and progression options of the seated upper-body resistance exercises (exercises 6.1–6.5) for instructions for the standing upper-body resistance exercises.

STANDING LOWER-BODY RESISTANCE AND BALANCE EXERCISES

Instructions for the standing lower-body resistance and balance exercises appear in the variations and progression options of the seated lower-body resistance exercises (exercises 6.6–6.12). As participants first learn the standing lower-body exercises, instruct them to hold on firmly to a secure support, such as the back of a steady chair or railing. To promote balance, participants should follow this progression:

1. Hold on firmly with two hands to a secure support.
2. Hold on gently with two hands.
3. Hold on firmly with one hand.
4. Hold on gently with one hand.
5. Hold on gently with four fingers, then three, then two, then one.
6. Do not hold on. If you lose your balance, have support within easy reach.

After participants have learned the exercises, they can move on to step 2. Those who are ready can slowly progress through the steps. Step 6 is only for those who are very steady on their feet and may not be appropriate with some of the exercises. It is easier to concentrate on a standing exercise while holding on to a support. If participants are unsteady during an exercise, help them find the grip that enables them to feel steady on their feet and perform the exercise comfortably. This support progression can also be applied when appropriate to standing range-of-motion (chapter 4) and stretching exercises (chapter 7).

TABLE 6.5 BASIC STANDING RESISTANCE AND BALANCE EXERCISES

Target body parts and major muscles	Standing upper-body resistance exercises	Functional role[a]	Page
Chest (pectoralis major) Back of upper arms (triceps) Shoulders (deltoids)	*6.1 Standing Chest Press	Pushing a door open, pushing up from a lying position, improved static standing balance	135
Back (latissimus dorsi, trapezius) Front of upper arms (biceps) Shoulders (deltoids)	*6.2 Standing Two-Arm Row	Pulling a door open, posture, improved static standing balance	137
Shoulders (deltoids) Back of upper arms (triceps)	*6.3 Standing Overhead Press	Lifting (especially overhead), improved static standing balance	138
Front of upper arms (biceps)	6.4 Standing Biceps Curl	Lifting, pulling, improved static standing balance	139
Back of upper arms (triceps)	6.5 Standing Triceps Extension (challenger)	Pushing, pressing up from seated or lying position, improved static standing balance	140

Target body parts and major muscles	Standing lower-body resistance exercises	Functional role[a]	Page
Thighs (quadriceps, hamstrings) Buttocks (gluteals)	*6.6 Chair Stands (challenger)	Stand from sitting, stair climbing, walking (forward progression and stability), improved static and dynamic standing balance	142
Front hips and thighs (hip flexors)	*6.7 Standing Hip Flexion	Stair climbing, posture, pelvic tilt, improved static and dynamic standing balance	143
Outer hips and thighs (hip abductors) Inner thighs (hip adductors)	*6.8 Standing Hip Abduction and Adduction	Hip rotation (lateral or medial), pelvic stabilization, posture, walking, improved static and dynamic standing balance	145
Back of thighs (hamstrings)	6.9 Standing Knee Flexion	Walking (foot clearance), improved static and dynamic standing balance	147
Front of thighs (quadriceps)	6.10 Standing Knee Extension	Stand from sitting, stair climbing, walking (forward progression and stability), improved static and dynamic standing balance	148
Shins (tibialis anterior)	*6.11 Standing Toe Raises	Walking (foot clearance), improved static and dynamic standing balance	149
Calves (gastrocnemius)	*6.12 Standing Heel Raises	Walking (push off), improved static and dynamic standing balance	150

[a]Adapted, by permission, from S. McKelvey, 2003, *Functional fitness for older adults training manual* (San Diego, CA: Aging and Independent Services) 7.

*The eight exercises preceded by an asterisk are recommended for a shorter program.

Variations and Progression

The section "Illustrated Resistance-Training Instruction" at the end of the chapter gives variations and progression options for each basic seated resistance exercise. You can introduce one or more of these variations after your participants have learned the basic seated exercises. The ability for extensive progression may be limited in some classes (e.g., a large class without an assistant in a long-term care setting), but varying the basic seated exercises can add spice to your class. Other classes may outgrow the seated exercises and be able to do a standing resistance workout. The variations and progression options enable you to design a creative and progressive fitness program that meets participants' needs.

The most important progression option is the standing exercises. Standing exercises offer participants the greatest benefits in functional mobility and increased independence. Each basic seated exercise has a standing alternative. The benefits of the standing variations and when the seated version is preferred are discussed in chapter 8.

There are countless ways of varying and progressing an exercise program. For example, since back muscles are prone to weakness, it can be worthwhile to do one set of the basic Seated Two-Arm Row and another set with an underhand-grip variation. For many other ideas for varying and progressing your class, see chapter 8.

SUMMARY

It is a common myth that seniors are too old to lift weights. In fact, people of all ages can benefit from appropriate resistance training. This chapter gives you simple guidelines, safety precautions, and teaching instructions for leading resistance exercises.

Following the safety precautions for resistance training helps to keep participants of any age injury-free. For example, keep blood pressure down by avoiding excessive amounts of overhead exercise, breath holding, and isometric exercises. The guidelines for beneficial results are two to three sessions per week on nonconsecutive days, a minimum of eight safe exercises that condition the major muscle groups of the body, and one to three sets of 8 to 15 repetitions of each exercise. Begin with the basic seated resistance exercises without weights. When participants have learned the exercises, begin with light weights; slowly progress. Participants who regularly resistance-train in your class can potentially have spectacular results, improving health, fitness, and performance of daily tasks.

Illustrated Resistance-Training Instruction

Exercises 6.1 to 6.5 are upper-body resistance exercises, and exercises 6.6 to 6.12 are lower-body resistance exercises. The "Exercise and Safety Tips" and "Variations and Progression Options" apply to both seated and standing exercises unless otherwise specified. The standing exercises and other variations and progression options that need further explanation are accompanied by a photograph and description.

SEATED CHEST PRESS

Target Muscles Chest (pectoralis major), back of upper arms (triceps), shoulders (deltoids)

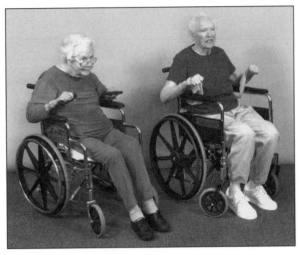

A

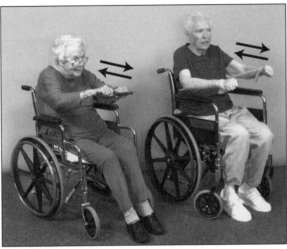

B

START/FINISH POSITION

1. Good seated posture.*
2. Upper arms by sides.
3. Hold weights with palms facing downward at level of lower chest.
4. Wrists straight.

OUTWARD/INWARD MOVEMENT

5. On the outward movement, count "1, 1, 1, out" or exhale.
6. On the inward movement, count "1, 1, 1, in" or inhale (return to start/finish position).
7. Move only elbow and shoulder joint.
8. Perform 8 to 12 repetitions.

Exercise and Safety Tips

- Stabilize shoulders (move them up, back, and down) before starting. Keep shoulders down.
- Keep wrists neutral (straight) during all upper-body resistance exercises, particularly when using bands and tubes.

Variations and Progression Options

- Modification: Upper arms may be held at a lower level if participants experience shoulder pain or fatigue, or just for variety.
- Chest Press combined with scapular retraction (squeezing shoulder blades together). Draw elbows backward toward each other.
- Standing Chest Press.
- Prop: Use a resistance band or tube for a more effective chest and triceps exercise. See appendix I, "Exercise Equipment," Resistance Bands and Tubes section.

Please note that the models in the photographs were unable to perform the chest press through the full ROM—straight arms and soft, unlocked elbows.

*See "Instructions for Good Seated Posture," page 63.

SEATED TWO-ARM ROW

Target Muscles   Back (latissimus dorsi, trapezius), front upper arms (biceps), shoulders (deltoids)

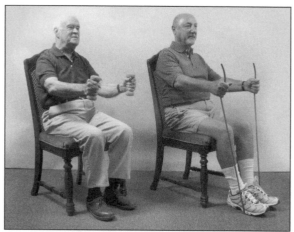

A

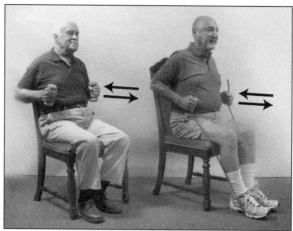

B

START/FINISH POSITION

1. Good seated posture.*
2. Arms straight out in front, slightly below shoulder level.
3. Hold weights or band with palms facing inward.

INWARD/OUTWARD MOVEMENT

4. On the inward movement, count "1, 1, 1, in" or exhale.
5. On the outward movement, count "1, 1, 1, out" or inhale (return to start/finish position).
6. Move only elbow and shoulder joint.
7. Perform 8 to 12 repetitions.

Exercise and Safety Tips

- Stabilize shoulders (move them up, back, and down) before starting. Keep them down.
- Move elbows straight backward, not to the side.
- On the backward rowing motion, gently squeeze shoulder blades together by drawing elbows toward one another behind your back.
- Keep wrists straight during all upper-body resistance exercises, particularly when using bands and tubes.
- Modification: If it can be done safely, move forward toward the middle of the chair so that elbows clear the back of the chair.

*See "Instructions for Good Seated Posture," page 63.

Variations and Progression Options

- Row with a narrow or wide grip.
- Row with an underhand or overhand grip.
- Modification: Upper arms can be held at a lower level if participants experience shoulder pain or fatigue, or just for variety.
- Prop: Use a resistance band or tube for a more effective back and biceps exercise. See appendix I, "Exercise Equipment," Resistance Bands and Tubes section.
- Standing Two-Arm Row (see photographs C and D and instructions).

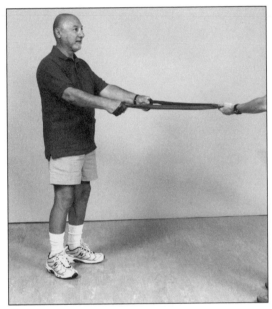

C

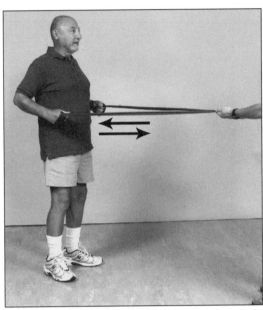

D

START/FINISH POSITION

1. Good standing posture.
2. Arms straight out in front, slightly below shoulder level.
3. Palms (with band) facing inward.

INWARD/OUTWARD MOVEMENT

4. Same as Seated Two-Arm Row.

SEATED OVERHEAD PRESS

Target Muscles   Shoulders (deltoids), back of upper arms (triceps)

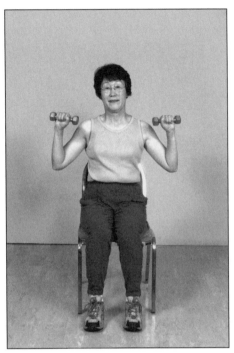

A

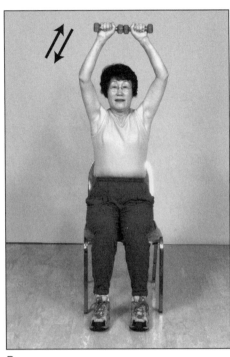

B

START/FINISH POSITION

1. Good seated posture.*
2. Hold weights at shoulder level.
3. Palms facing forward.

UPWARD/DOWNWARD MOVEMENT

4. On the upward movement, count "1, 1, 1, up" or exhale.
5. On the downward movement, count "1, 1, 1, down" or inhale (return to start/finish position).
6. Move only the shoulder and elbow joint.
7. Perform 8 to 12 repetitions.

Exercise and Safety Tips

- Lift the weights in front of the head, as if lifting an object onto a high shelf.
- Modification: If participants experience any strain or pain in the shoulder joints when doing the Overhead Press, they should not lift the weights as high.

Variations and Progression Options

- When a participant is unable to lift the weight through the full range of motion, he or she should gradually over time reach higher, always within their *pain-free* range of motion.
- Standing Overhead Press.

*See "Instructions for Good Seated Posture," page 63.

SEATED BICEPS CURL

Target Muscles Front of upper arms (biceps)

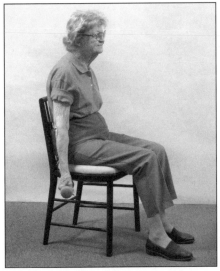

A

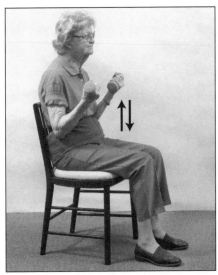

B

START/FINISH POSITION

1. Good seated posture.*
2. Arms down at sides, upper arms touch sides of torso.
3. Hold weights with palms facing forward.

UPWARD/DOWNWARD MOVEMENT

4. On the upward movement, count "1, 1, 1, up" or exhale.
5. On the downward movement, count "1, 1, 1, down" or inhale (return to start/finish position).
6. Move only elbow joint.
7. Perform 8 to 12 repetitions.

! Exercise and Safety Tips

- Stabilize shoulders (move them up, back, and down) before starting. Keep them down.
- Avoid leaning to one side when performing the Biceps Curl on one side.
- Upper arms remain stationary ("glued to your side") throughout the Biceps Curl.
- Modification: If the chair has arms, move forward toward the middle of the chair if it is safe to do so, so that the elbows clear the chair arms.
- Check participants' posture to be sure they are not leaning backward, especially when they are sitting in the middle of their chairs or standing.

Variations and Progression Options

- Perform Biceps Curl with one arm at a time, a good way to start.
- Perform Biceps Curl with palms facing each other (inward) throughout the exercise, a Hammer Curl, or facing backward (in the starting position).
- Standing Biceps Curl or Standing Hammer Curl.

*See "Instructions for Good Seated Posture," page 63.

SEATED TRICEPS EXTENSION (CHALLENGER)

Target Muscles   Back of upper arms (triceps)

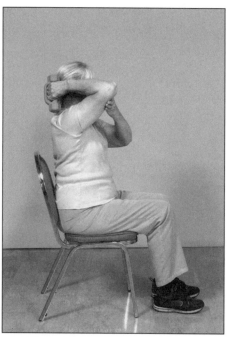

A

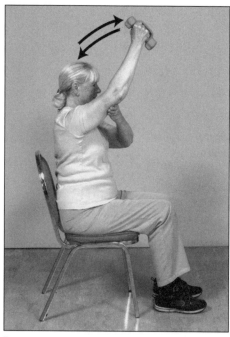

B

START/FINISH POSITION

1. Good seated posture.*
2. Hold weight with palm facing inward.
3. Lift upper arm as high as comfortable.
4. Hold back of upper arm with opposite hand.

UPWARD/DOWNWARD MOVEMENT

5. On the upward movement, count "1, 1, 1, up" or exhale.
6. On the downward movement, count "1, 1, 1, down" or inhale (return to start/finish position).
7. Move only elbow joint.
8. Perform 8 to 12 repetitions.
9. Repeat on other side.

Exercise and Safety Tips

- Stabilize shoulders (move them up, back, and down) before starting. Keep them down.
- Keep the working upper arm as high as possible while maintaining good posture.
- The upper arm (of the working triceps) remains stationary throughout the Triceps Extension.
- Check participants' postures to be sure they are not leaning backward.

Variations and Progression Options

- Stretch the triceps (see exercise 7.5, Zipper Stretch, in chapter 7) before doing the Triceps Extension.
- Standing Triceps Extension.

*See "Instructions for Good Seated Posture," page 63.

MODIFIED CHAIR STANDS (CHALLENGER)

Target Muscles   Thighs (quadriceps, hamstrings), buttocks (gluteals)

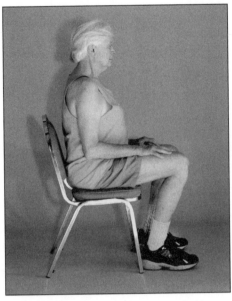

A

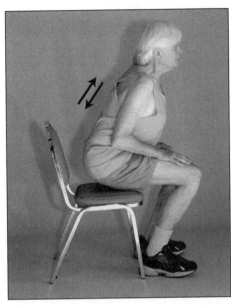

B

START/FINISH POSITION

1. Good seated posture.*
2. Palms on thighs.
3. Feet hip-width apart.

UPWARD/DOWNWARD MOVEMENT

4. On the upward movement, count "1, 1, 1, up" or exhale.
5. On the downward movement, count "1, 1, 1, down" or inhale (return to start/finish position).
6. Move only hip, knee, and ankle joint.
7. Perform 8 to 12 repetitions.

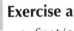

Exercise and Safety Tips

- *Spot* (one-on-one facilitation) those with balance problems.
- Keep shoulders down throughout the exercise.
- Lean forward from the hips, and push off thighs with hands while standing.
- Start by raising the buttocks 1 inch (2.5 centimeters) off the chair, then slowly sit back down. Do 8 to 15 repetitions.
- Maintain a neutral spine (see figure 4.2). Move head, neck, and spine as one unit.
- Do not project the knees beyond the toes in any weight-bearing exercise.
- Remind those with knee problems to stay within their pain-free range of motion, even if that range is quite limited.

(continued)

*See "Instructions for Good Seated Posture," page 63.

(continued)

Variations and Progression Options

- Props: Push off using the seat or arms of the chair, a cane, or a walker (with brake on).
- Use hand weights when participants are ready to make Chair Stands more challenging. Without weights, put arms in a comfortable position, such as crossed across chest.
- Chair Stands (challenger) (see photographs C and D and instructions).

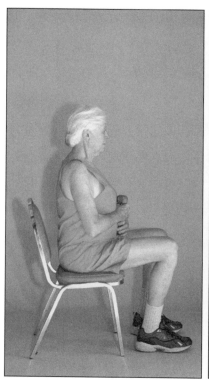 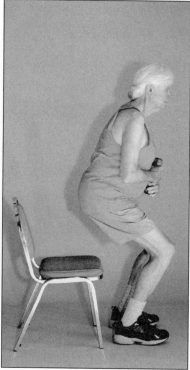 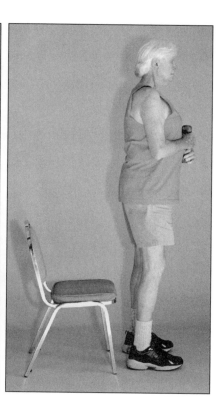

C   **D**

START/FINISH POSITION

1. Good seated posture.*
2. Hold weights with palms facing chest.
3. Rest hands on chest.
4. Feet shoulder-width apart.

UPWARD/DOWNWARD MOVEMENT

5. Same as Modified Chair Stands.

*See "Instructions for Good Seated Posture," page 63.

SEATED HIP FLEXION

Target Muscles   Front hips and thighs (hip flexors)

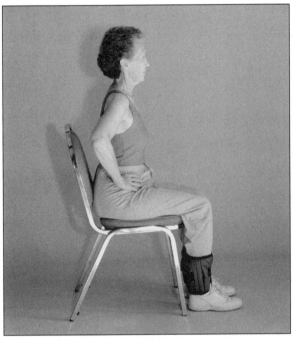

A

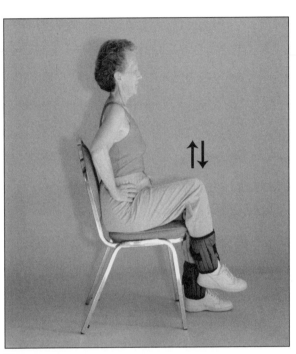

B

START/FINISH POSITION

1. Good seated posture.*
2. Hands on hips.

UPWARD/DOWNWARD MOVEMENT

3. On the upward movement, count "1, 1, 1, up" or exhale.
4. On the downward movement, count "1, 1, 1, down" or inhale (return to start/finish position).
5. Move only hip joint.
6. Perform 8 to 12 repetitions.
7. Repeat on other side.

Exercise and Safety Tips

- Lift the legs only as high as comfortable while maintaining erect posture.
- Feel hip flexors working.

Variations and Progression Options

- Lift leg higher.
- Standing Hip Flexion.

*See "Instructions for Good Seated Posture," page 63.

SEATED HIP ABDUCTION AND ADDUCTION

Target Muscles   Outer hips and thighs (hip abductors), inner thighs (hip adductors)

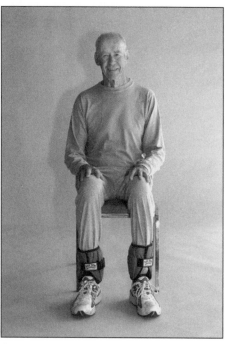

A

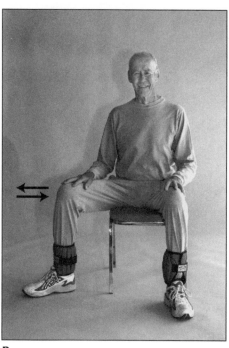

B

START/FINISH POSITION

1. Good seated posture.*
2. Hands in comfortable position.

OUTWARD/INWARD MOVEMENT

3. On the outward movement, count "1, 1, 1, out" or exhale.
4. On the inward movement, count "1, 1, 1, in" or inhale (return to start/finish position).
5. Move only the hip joint.
6. Perform 8 to 12 repetitions.
7. Repeat on other side.

Exercise and Safety Tips

- When seated, keep each foot directly below each knee.
- When standing, keep toes of moving foot pointed straight ahead.
- When adducting the leg (inward movement) while standing, cross the midline of the body as far as comfortable, keeping the torso stationary.

*See "Instructions for Good Seated Posture," page 63.

Variations and Progression Options

- Lift leg while abducting and adducting in seated position, similar to the motion of lifting a leg in and out of a car. This variation is contraindicated for those who have had hip replacement surgery, who should avoid flexing the hip more than 90 degrees.
- Standing Hip Abduction and Adduction (see photographs C and D and instructions).

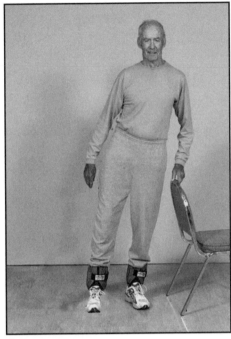

C

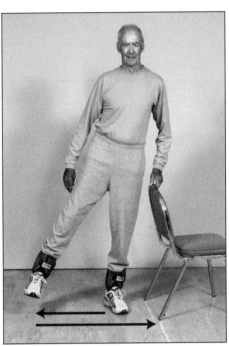

D

START/FINISH POSITION

1. Good standing posture.
2. Hold on to a secure support with one hand.

OUTWARD/INWARD MOVEMENT

3. Same as Seated Hip Abduction and Adduction.
4. On the inward movement, the moving leg crosses the midline.

SEATED KNEE FLEXION

Target Muscles   Back of thighs (hamstrings)

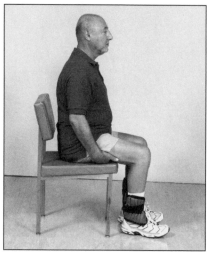

A

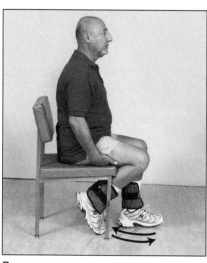

B

START/FINISH POSITION

1. Good seated posture.*
2. Hands under thighs.

UPWARD/DOWNWARD MOVEMENT

3. On the upward movement, count "1, 1, 1, up" or exhale.
4. On the downward movement, count "1, 1, 1, down" or inhale (return to start/finish position).
5. Move only knee joint.
6. Perform 8 to 12 repetitions.
7. Repeat on other side.

Exercise and Safety Tips

- Feel hamstrings working.
- Modification: If bars between the front legs of the chairs impede movement, instruct participants to move forward 4 to 6 inches (10–15 centimeters) in their seats if they can do so safely. Instruct them to hold on to the sides or arms of their chairs when sitting forward in their chairs.
- During Standing Knee Flexion, keep knees aligned.

Variations and Progression Options

- Bring the heel up higher but still within a pain-free range of motion.
- Standing Knee Flexion (see photographs C and D and instructions on the next page).

*See "Instructions for Good Seated Posture," page 63.

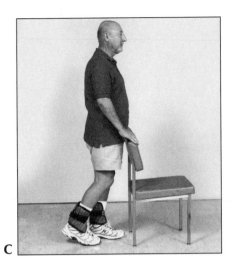

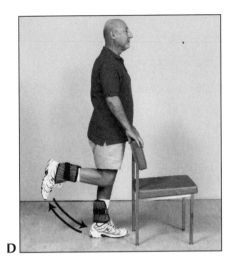

C

START/FINISH POSITION

1. Good standing posture.
2. Hands holding on to a secure support.
3. Knee slightly bent.

D

UPWARD/DOWNWARD MOVEMENT

4. Same as Seated Knee Flexion.

| LOWER-BODY RESISTANCE EXERCISES | EXERCISE 6.10 |

SEATED KNEE EXTENSION

Target Muscles   Front thighs (quadriceps)

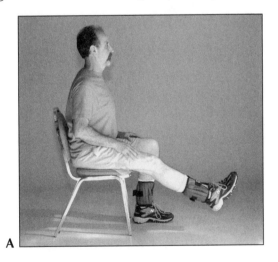

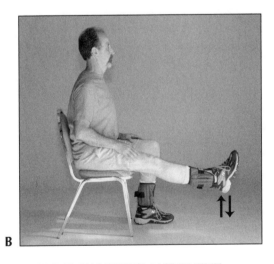

A

B

START/FINISH POSITION

1. Good seated posture.*
2. Palms on thighs.
3. Leg slightly bent.

UPWARD/DOWNWARD MOVEMENT

4. On the upward movement, count "1, 1, 1, up" or exhale.
5. On the downward movement, count "1, 1, 1, down" or inhale (return to start/finish position).
6. Move only knee joint.
7. Perform 8 to 12 repetitions.
8. Repeat on other side.

*See "Instructions for Good Seated Posture," page 63.

(continued)

(continued)

Exercise and Safety Tips

- Feel quadriceps working.
- Avoid extending the knee through the full range of motion when using leg weights, which can cause the back of the *patella* (knee cap) to degenerate.
- After initially straightening the leg, lower it only 6 inches (15 centimeters).
- Scoot buttocks all the way to the back of the chair for maximum back support.
- When standing, the working thigh can be raised less than 90 degrees.

Variations and Progression Options

- Stretch the hamstrings (exercise 7.8, Tib Touches, in chapter 7) before doing the Standing Knee Extension. As their hamstring flexibility increases, standing participants will be able to lift the thigh higher than 45 degrees.
- Plantar flex (point the toes) and then dorsiflex (toes toward nose) the ankle with each repetition when leg is straight.
- Standing Knee Extension (see photographs C and D and instructions).

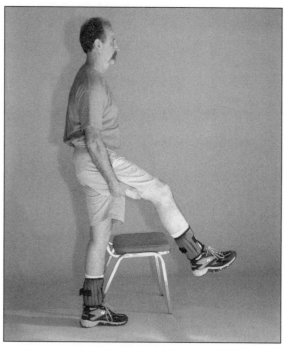

C
START/FINISH POSITION

1. Good standing posture.
2. Hold on to a secure support with one hand.
3. One thigh at 45 degrees.
4. Same leg slightly bent.
5. Support thigh with hand.

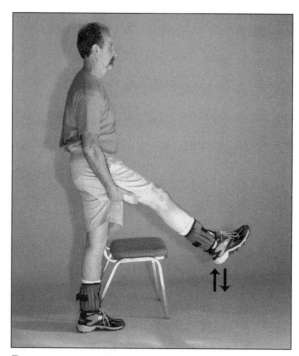

D
UPWARD/DOWNWARD MOVEMENT

6. Same as Seated Knee Extension.

SEATED TOE RAISES

Target Muscles   Shins (tibialis anterior)

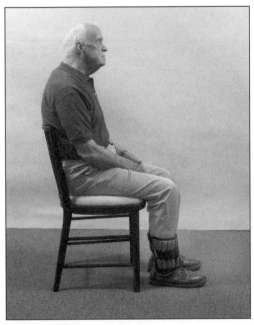

A

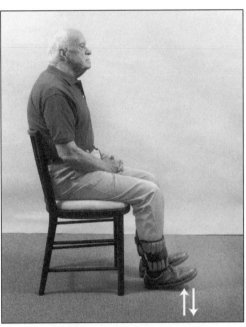

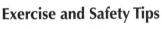

B

START/FINISH POSITION

1. Good seated posture.*
2. Hands in comfortable position.

UPWARD/DOWNWARD MOVEMENT

3. On the upward movement, count "1, 1, 1, up" or exhale.
4. On the downward movement, count "1, 1, 1, down" or inhale (return to start/finish position).
5. Move only ankle joint.
6. Perform 8 to 12 repetitions.

!

Exercise and Safety Tips

- Instruct participants to not rock the whole body back when raising their toes. Focus on moving only the ankle joint.

Variations and Progression Options

- Standing Toe Raises.
- Prop: Use a wall to support the upper body during Standing Toe Raises.

*See "Instructions for Good Seated Posture," page 63.

SEATED HEEL RAISES

Target Muscles   Calves (gastrocnemius, soleus)

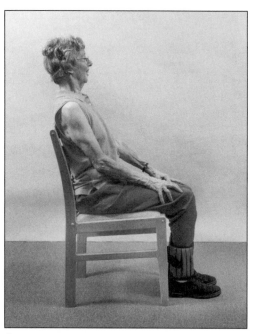

A

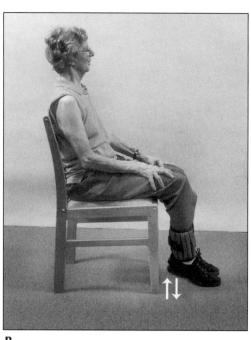

B

START/FINISH POSITION

1. Good seated posture.*
2. Hands in comfortable position.

UPWARD/DOWNWARD MOVEMENT

3. On the upward movement, count "1, 1, 1, up" or exhale.
4. On the downward movement, count "1, 1, 1, down" or inhale (return to start/finish position).
5. Move only ankle joint.
6. Perform 8 to 12 repetitions.

Exercise and Safety Tips

- Instruct participants to distribute their weight evenly on the balls of the feet when the heels are lifted.

Variations and Progression Options

- One-legged heel raises.
- Standing Heel Raises.

*See "Instructions for Good Seated Posture," page 63.

CHAPTER 7

Cool-Down: Stretching and Relaxation Exercises

This chapter provides guidelines, safety precautions, and teaching instructions for the cooling-down period after exercise. Stopping exercise abruptly creates a risk of irregular heartbeat, dizziness, fainting, and coughing and wheezing for those with asthma and bronchitis. Always have your participants cool down to facilitate the transition between exercise and rest and to promote *flexibility* (the ability to move joints and muscles through their full, normal range of motion) and relaxation. The cool-down consists of slow, controlled movements that slowly lower the heart rate and stretching exercises. This is also an ideal time for leading relaxation exercises.

The stretching and relaxation exercises in this chapter can help you lead a safe and effective cool-down. Start with the basic seated stretching exercises. Participants who are able to stand safely can carefully progress to the basic standing stretching exercises. The seated and standing exercises are designed to be taught together to accommodate both those who can stand and those who cannot or who prefer to sit.

Safety Precautions for Cool-Down Exercises

The following general safety precautions and specific safety precautions for those with special needs can help you lead a safe cool-down. You may photocopy the following "General Safety Precautions Checklist for Stretching" and the general exercise "Safety Guidelines Checklist" in chapter 2.

Specific Safety Precautions for Those With Special Needs

Following are some safety precautions for leading the cool-down for those with special needs. They may not apply to every individual with a particular condition. For example, an individual with mild symptoms of Parkinson's disease may have no limitations on stretching exercises, whereas severe symptoms may cause difficulty with all stretching exercises. Also, remember that individuals' performance abilities can vary from day to day. See chapter 1 to learn more about common medical disorders in the elderly. Above all, follow the physician's or physical therapist's special exercise recommendations for the participant.

Arthritis

- A thorough cool-down is especially important for individuals with arthritis, whose joints need extra time to recover from extended periods of exercise.

General Safety Precautions Checklist for Stretching

❑ Review the physician's or physical therapist's comments and special recommendations for each participant on the medical clearance form.

❑ Remind participants to observe recommendations from their physicians or physical therapists.

❑ Always leave at least 10 minutes at the end of class for a cool-down period. Cool-down exercises done right after exercise reduce the incidence of cardiovascular complications (Balady et al. 2000, 143).

❑ Do not move a joint beyond its pain-free range of motion.

❑ Avoid hyperextending (locking) any joints when stretching.

❑ Avoid stretching beyond the body's natural limits. Overstretching weakens joints and increases risk of injury (Picone 2000, 378).

❑ Always keep one foot planted firmly on the floor while stretching the other leg to help prevent lower-back strain.

❑ Remind participants to stop deep breathing if they feel light-headed or dizzy.

❑ Continually encourage your participants to maintain good posture and breathing (no breath holding) while exercising and throughout the day.

❑ Focus on fun and safety!

From *Exercise for Frail Elders* by E. Best-Martini and K. A. Botenhagen-DiGenova, 2003, Champaign, IL: Human Kinetics.

- Stretching is recommended once to several times a day. Encourage a safe home program for those who are capable.

CEREBROVASCULAR ACCIDENT (STROKE)

- The American Senior Fitness Association (2003a, 18) recommends that people with a history of stroke hold neck stretches no longer than 2 to 3 seconds. No longer than 5 seconds is recommended for elderly participants in general.

- Always keep the head above the heart when bending forward, because of the danger of increased vascular pressure within the brain and the risk of stroke. We have excluded such exercises from this book. We suggest that stroke survivors, those at risk for stroke, and those with glaucoma pay particular attention to this precaution when bending forward to tie shoes, pick up weights from the floor, and so on.

CHRONIC OBSTRUCTIVE PULMONARY DISEASE

- A thorough cool-down is critical for individuals with COPD, whose lungs and cardiovascular systems need extra time to adapt to changes in exertion level.

CORONARY ARTERY DISEASE (HEART DISEASE)

- A careful cool-down is critical for participants with heart disease, whose cardiovascular systems need extra time to adapt to changes in exertion level.

DIABETES

- People with peripheral vascular disease (which causes poor circulation to the legs and feet), to which people with diabetes are predisposed, should avoid crossed-leg positions when stretching, as in exercise 7.11, Seated Outer-Thigh Stretch.

HIP FRACTURE OR REPLACEMENT

- Avoid stretching exercises that involve internal rotation (turning the leg inward), hip adduction (crossing the legs), and hip flexion greater than 90 degrees (thigh higher than parallel with floor) to prevent the risk of hip dislocation. A safe modification of the Seated or Standing Tib Touches (exercise 7.8) for a participant with a hip replacement who is good at following directions is to do them while seated without leaning forward. Do the Seated or Standing Outer-Thigh Stretch (exercise 7.11) without crossing the legs.

MULTIPLE SCLEROSIS AND PARKINSON'S DISEASE

- Stretching is recommended five to seven times per week.
- If you cannot offer classes that often, encourage a home program for those who are capable.
- When working one-on-one with individuals who have both coordination and flexibility limitations, consider functional flexibility exercises, such as using a stationary bicycle. Such exercises may serve better than standard stretching, especially early in training.

- Anyone with any trouble controlling neck movement should avoid neck stretches because of the increased risk of injury.

OSTEOPOROSIS

- Stretching is recommended five to seven times per week. If you cannot offer class that often, encourage a home program for those who are capable.
- Avoid stretching exercises that involve spinal flexion (such as exercise 7.8, Tib Touches), particularly in combination with stooping, which increases risk of vertebral fractures. A safe adaptation for Seated and Standing Tib Touches for someone with osteoporosis who is good at following directions is to do them while seated without leaning forward.

SENSORY LOSSES

- Give a clear demonstration of the cool-down exercises to participants with hearing loss.
- Describe cool-down exercises precisely and directly to participants with visual impairment.

GUIDELINES FOR COOL-DOWN EXERCISES

The cool-down exercises in this chapter focus on flexibility and relaxation. A comprehensive set of stretches and some simple relaxation exercises are given. Leave at least 10 minutes at the end of your class for the cool-down. Table 7.1 shows duration of the parts of a 10- to 15-minute cool-down segment.

TABLE 7.1 DURATION OF THE SEGMENTS OF A 10- TO 15-MINUTE COOL-DOWN

Cool-down exercises[a]	After aerobics	After resistance training
1. Low-level aerobics	5 minutes[b]	Not applicable
2. Range-of-motion exercises	1 to 3 minutes	3 minutes
3. Stretching	3 to 5 minutes	6 to 7 minutes
4. Relaxation	1 to 2 minutes	1 to 5 minutes

[a]Exercises are in the recommended order.
[b]Times are approximate.

Notice that the cool-down following aerobics includes low-level aerobics: progressively slower-paced movements that allow the respiration rate, heart rate, and blood pressure to gradually decrease to the pre-aerobic state. See chapter 5 for aerobic exercises that can be performed slowly at a lower intensity. The cool-down phase after resistance training begins with range-of-motion exercises (see chapter 4) and concentrates on stretching. Range-of-motion exercises consist of gentle movements that gradually lower the breathing, heart rate, and blood pressure.

The following sections present guidelines for stretching and relaxation exercises that apply to both seated and standing exercises.

Guidelines for Stretching Exercises

A well-rounded stretching program can prevent or even reverse the usual decline in flexibility of older adults and improve their posture, balance, and functional ability. As participants' flexibility improves, they can more easily perform daily activities requiring flexibility, such as bathing, grooming, dressing and undressing, reaching, and so on. Several prominent organizations have developed guidelines for stretching, including the American College of Sports Medicine (1998a, 1998b), the American Council on Exercise (Cotton et al. 1998), the American Senior Fitness Association (2003b), the National Strength

and Conditioning Association (Earle and Baechle 2000), and the YMCA of the USA (2000). Table 7.2 synthesizes the stretching guidelines that are appropriate for older adults. The basic seated and standing stretching exercises in this chapter are based on these well-researched guidelines. You may make a copy of table 7.2 for easy reference and as an educational handout for your participants.

When to Stretch During a Workout

The best time to improve long-term flexibility is at the end of a workout, when muscles are warm and pliable. Cool down a minimum of 10 minutes after aerobics and resistance training (see table 7.1 for the components and duration of the cool-down). If you are leading both aerobics and resistance training in one class, with aerobics before resistance training, finish with several minutes of low-intensity aerobic exercise using the legs. Follow this with the minimal five stretching exercises (see table 4.3 in chapter 4) before you begin resistance training. If you do resistance exercises before aerobics, do the minimal five stretches, and then perform several minutes of active rhythmic movement (such as slow walking or low-intensity aerobic leg exercises) before starting aerobic work. After aerobics, cool down with several minutes of low-intensity aerobic exercise and range-of-motion exercises before stretching.

Light stretching is done at the end of the warm-up, before aerobics or resistance exercises (refer to

TABLE 7.2	General Stretching Guidelines for Older Adults
When to stretch during a workout	At the end of the warm-up before exercise, and after exercise. If you do both aerobics and resistance training in one class, also briefly stretch between those components.
Frequency	Two to seven times per week
Exercise selection	Stretch the major muscle groups of the body.
Stretching mode	Static stretching is recommended over ballistic stretching.
Intensity (how should a stretch feel)	Stretches should be taken only to the point of tightness or mild intensity, not pain.
Duration (how long to hold a stretch)	10 to 30 seconds, except 5 seconds or less for neck stretches
Number of times to repeat a stretch	1 to 5
Speed	Slowly ease in and out of a stretch.
Rest periods between sets of the same stretch	A few seconds
Rest periods between different stretches	None to a few seconds

From *Exercise for Frail Elders* by E. Best-Martini and K. A. Botenhagen-DiGenova, 2003, Champaign, IL: Human Kinetics.

table 4.1, chapter 4). If you are teaching a stretching-only class, warm up for a minimum of 10 minutes beforehand to increase circulation, internal body temperature, and joint range of motion.

FREQUENCY

Since flexibility and freedom of movement typically decline with age, older adults can greatly benefit from a regular stretching program. Ideally, they should participate in a fitness class that includes stretching more often than the recommended minimum of twice per week. Two to three days per week of stretching is considered a maintenance program. For progression, five to seven days per week of stretching are recommended. On the days that you do not offer stretching, encourage your participants to stretch on their own (if they are able) after they have learned the stretches in class. The minimal five stretching exercises (table 4.3) and the short-routine eight stretches (table 4.4) are ideal for an independent program. You may copy these tables for your participants.

EXERCISE SELECTION

Stretching-only classes should include an initial warm-up period of light movement (see chapter 4), the stretching exercises, and a final period of relaxation. The comprehensive stretching session in this chapter includes seven upper-body and five lower-body basic stretches that target the major muscle groups of the body. These exercises are safe and appropriate for frail elders and adults with special needs.

For a shorter set of stretching exercises see table 4.3, "The Minimal Five Stretching Exercises," or table 4.4, "Eight Warm-Up Stretches," in chapter 4. These shorter stretching sessions both include essential stretches for body parts that are notoriously tight for the majority of older adults and that can compromise posture, impair balance, and reduce functional ability. These shorter sessions are derived from the comprehensive stretching exercises. No matter how many stretching exercises you do, start with the basic seated stretches. Participants who are stable on their feet can progress to basic standing stretching exercises.

STRETCHING MODE

Static (held or sustained) stretching is a simple, effective, and safe method, so long as it is not done too strenuously. Conversely, ballistic stretching—high-force, short-duration bouncing, jerking, or swinging motion—is not recommended because it is less effective than static stretching and carries a greater risk of injuring muscles and connective tissue. The preferred static stretch is slow and constant with the end or stretch position (the position that stretches the muscle to the greatest length) held without movement for 10 to 30 seconds.

INTENSITY

Instruct participants to stretch only to the point of tightness or a pulling sensation of mild intensity, not to the point of strain or pain. Slowly stretch as far as possible into this end position. With each stretch, remind participants to breathe, relax, and focus on lengthening (or "letting go of") the muscles involved in the stretch. A stretch should be felt in the muscle and not the joint. Minimize movement of body parts that are not involved in the stretch.

How do you know whether a participant is stretching effectively?

- If they do not feel the stretch, they have not gone far enough.
- If they feel the stretch, a mild tightness, they have gone far enough.
- If they feel pain, they have gone too far. In this case, reduce the stretch so that it does not hurt.

When describing how a stretch should feel to your participants, use positive words, such as "pleasant pulling sensation," to describe the end point rather than "mild discomfort" or other terms with negative connotations.

DURATION

The recommended duration for a stretch is 10 to 30 seconds, depending on the muscle or muscles being stretched, the individual's tolerance, and the time available. However, hold neck stretches for 5 seconds or less. Encourage participants to hold a stretch for only as long as it feels comfortable. In other words, each participant should stop a stretch when he or she feels tired or uncomfortable and resume the stretch when he or she feels ready, regardless of what the rest of the class is doing. A good long-term goal is to gradually build up to sustaining each stretch for 30 seconds. You can time stretches silently with a clock or stopwatch rather than counting aloud for a quieter, more relaxing atmosphere.

NUMBER OF TIMES TO REPEAT A STRETCH

A realistic number of times to repeat a stretch is one to five times. If you are short on time at the end of class, do a stretch once slowly with concentration. For optimal flexibility gains, leave enough time at the end of class to repeat each stretch at least three times.

When performing additional stretches, stretch the muscles in various positions when possible. For example, with the Swan stretch (exercise 7.3), hold the arms at various heights from parallel with the floor to at one's sides. Stretching in different positions can enhance muscle relaxation and improve range of motion of the joints.

SPEED

Move slowly and smoothly in and out of a stretch. Coach your participants to breathe and move gracefully from one repetition of the same stretch to another and between different stretches.

REST PERIODS

Rest a few seconds between repetitions of the same stretch. You can also rest a few seconds between different stretches or flow from one stretch to the next. Rest periods can be longer if you are leading a stretching-only class. Rest periods are a good time to do two-part deep breathing (chapter 4), a range-of-motion exercise (chapter 4), take a drink of water, or gently shake out the arms or legs that were stretched.

OTHER STRETCHING TECHNIQUES

- Participants should wear clothing that does not restrict movement.
- Participants should avoid hyperextending (overstretching or locking) the knee and elbow joints when straightening them during stretches. They should maintain a very small bend in the joints while stretching.
- If participants tend to lift their shoulders while stretching, have them stabilize their shoulders by moving them up, back, and down. Shoulders should be kept down.
- Participants should breathe slowly and deeply while holding the stretches and not hold their breath.
- Instruct participants to focus on or feel the major muscles that are being stretched.
- You should never apply force to participants while they are stretching.
- After each stretch, very gently shake out the area stretched to release any residual muscle tension. "This is especially important in the beginning stages, since the learning itself may set us up for the stress response" (Scheller 1993, 39).
- Have fun!

GUIDELINES FOR RELAXATION EXERCISES

By the time they reach the cool-down, your participants should be feeling more relaxed than before exercise; exercise is one of the best tools for stress reduction. An effective stretching program also promotes relaxation of mind and body. Adding a relaxation exercise to your cool-down can further contribute to a tranquil mood in your class and relieve participants' muscular tension and stress. Following are guidelines for leading relaxation exercises.

WHEN TO LEAD RELAXATION EXERCISES DURING A WORKOUT

The end of a fitness class is typically the best time to do relaxation exercises. Furthermore, you can conduct a fitness class with an emphasis on relaxation by integrating breathing into the workout. For instance, participants can deep-breathe between resistance exercises and during and between stretching exercises.

FREQUENCY

Relaxation exercises can be done one to seven times per week—the more, the better, as long as relaxation exercises are not taking the place of a well-rounded fitness program.

DURATION

You can lead a short relaxation exercise at the end of class, an entire relaxation class, or integrate relaxation into your exercise program when appropriate. If you only have a minute or less at the end of class, try one or two relaxing deep breaths. On the other hand, if you are dedicating an entire class to relaxation, you can use more than one relaxation exercise.

NUMBER OF TIMES TO REPEAT A RELAXATION EXERCISE

In a short relaxation segment at the end of class, you might do a relaxation exercise just once. However, breathing exercises can be repeated several times to fill the time available. With a relaxation-only class, you can do relaxation exercises several times. You can also creatively extend an exercise. A tried and true guided imagery technique is to invite participants to go to "a favorite, relaxing place."

SPEED

Proceed slowly. Never hurry through the relaxation exercise. This can cause a counterproductive stress response.

OTHER TRAINING TIPS

- Have your students perform the relaxation exercises while seated, not standing; sitting makes it easier to relax. If your participants practice any of the relaxation exercises at home, let them know that the exercises can also be done while lying down.

- Try to create a quiet, undistracting environment. After participants have learned to relax in silence, it can be beneficial to practice relaxation techniques under normal circumstances, such as while phones are ringing or with the television on in the background.

- Dim the lights for the relaxation exercises, if possible. To prevent falls, turn the lights back to normal before the participants get up.

- Relaxing music can enhance relaxation.

- You can record the verbal guidance for relaxation exercises involving guided imagery on audiotape for future use.

BASIC SEATED COOL-DOWN EXERCISES

The basic seated cool-down focuses on stretching and includes relaxation exercises. Begin teaching the basic seated cool-down exercises before the basic standing stretching exercises. We recommend that relaxation only be done seated. Participants who are able to stand safely can slowly progress to the basic standing stretching exercises. Before teaching these exercises, be sure to review the guidelines and safety precautions for cool-down exercises. If you are a new instructor or would like to refine your instructional skills, review the three-step instructional process (see chapter 3).

BASIC SEATED STRETCHING EXERCISES

The basic seated stretching exercises (table 7.3) are a comprehensive set of seven upper-body stretches

TABLE 7.3 BASIC SEATED STRETCHING EXERCISES

Target body parts and major muscles	Seated upper-body stretches	Page
Neck (neck extensors)	7.1 Seated Chin to Chest	161
Neck (neck rotators and extensors)	7.2 Seated Chin to Shoulder	162
Chest (pectoralis major) Shoulders (deltoids) Front upper arms (biceps)	m,s7.3 Seated Swan	163
Back (latissimus dorsi) Shoulders (deltoids)	7.4 Seated Half Hug	164
Back of upper arms (triceps) Back (latissimus dorsi)	m,s7.5 Seated Zipper Stretch	165
Side of torso (abdominals)	7.6 Seated Side Bends	166
Torso (abdominals, spinal erectors)	m,s7.7 Seated Spinal Twist	167
Target body parts and major muscles	Seated lower-body stretches	Page
Back of thighs (hamstrings) Back (spinal erectors)	m,s7.8 Seated Tib Touches	168
Front thighs (quadriceps) Shins (tibialis anterior)	s7.9 Seated Quad Stretch	169
Inner thighs (hip adductors)	s7.10 Seated Splits	171
Outer hips and thighs (hip abductors)	s7.11 Seated Outer-Thigh Stretch	172
Calves (gastrocnemius, soleus)	m,s7.12 Seated Calf Stretch	174

The five exercises preceded by an *m* are recommended for a minimal stretching routine. The eight exercises preceded by an *s* are recommended for a short stretching routine.

From *Exercise for Frail Elders* by E. Best-Martini and K. A. Botenhagen-DiGenova, 2003, Champaign, IL: Human Kinetics.

and five lower-body stretches. If you have only the minimal 10 minutes for the cool-down, start with a shorter stretching routine. Two shorter sets of seated stretching exercises appear in tables 4.3 and 4.4 in chapter 4. You may copy tables 7.3, 4.3, and 4.4 for easy reference.

Before leading the seated stretching exercises, note the following tips:

- Review the general exercise "Safety Guidelines Checklist" (in chapter 2) and the section "General Safety Precautions Checklist for Stretching" (earlier in this chapter) before leading these exercises.

- See the photographs, teaching instructions, and variations and progression options at the end of this chapter.

- Basic seated stretching exercises can be adapted to standing exercises. See the section "Basic Standing Stretching Exercises" later in this chapter.

Learn—and teach your participants—the body parts and major muscles addressed by each stretching exercise. This knowledge can help your participants focus on the body part or major muscles they are stretching. See appendix J, Muscles of the Human Body. You may make a copy of appendix J to refer to during class.

Basic Seated Relaxation Exercises

There is insubstantial evidence that one type of relaxation training is more effective than another. Following are some enjoyable relaxation exercises that include deep breathing and guided imagery. The "Suggested Resources" at the back of this book provide sources of additional relaxation techniques.

Deep Breathing

Breathing exercises are easy to learn and require little time. Teach your participants to practice deep breathing throughout the day for relaxation. Here are two breathing exercises:

1. Two-part deep-breathing (Scheller 1993). Instructions for the two-part deep-breathing exercise can be found in chapter 4. Teach this basic breathing exercise before introducing the next one.

2. Deep-breathing exercise. Inhale on a count of 4 to 8, hold for 1 count, exhale on a count of 4

to 8. This relaxation exercise is described in figure 7.1. After a few deep breaths, increase the exhale by one count, then two, and so on. A longer exhalation is relaxing and makes room in the lungs for a longer inhalation. Encourage participants to breathe at their own pace, never straining, especially those with COPD.

Guided Imagery

After participants are at ease with the breathing exercises, you can progress to combining imagery with deep breathing. The guided imagery with deep-breathing exercise (figure 7.1) is a multisensory relaxation exercise. Guided imagery is a form of autosuggestion or self-hypnosis that uses visual images to elicit a relaxation response. First, practice the deep-breathing exercise, then lead participants in either the one-step guided imagery or three-step guided imagery described in figure 7.1. If you choose the three-step guided imagery, start with steps 1 and 3. Watch how your class responds. When they are ready for more, add step 2. Be creative in conjuring up tranquil settings for step 2.

Basic Standing Stretching Exercises

The basic standing stretching exercises can replace the basic seated stretching exercises, or both can be taught at the same time. We recommend that anyone who cannot safely stand continue with the seated stretching exercises. Any participant with *minor* balance problems should perform only those standing exercises that leave a hand available to hold on to a secure support. Standing stretches that require two hands, such as the Swan, Half Hug, Zipper, and Spinal Twist, should be performed only by participants who are steady on their feet.

The basic standing stretching exercises (table 7.4) are a comprehensive set of seven upper-body stretches and five lower-body stretches. If you only have the minimal 10 minutes for the cool-down period, start with one of the shorter stretching routines (see tables 4.3 and 4.4 in chapter 4).

Before leading the standing stretching exercises, note the following tips:

- Start with the basic seated stretching exercises.

GUIDED IMAGERY WITH DEEP-BREATHING EXERCISE

Deep-Breathing Exercise

Do this deep breathing exercise before the guided imagery exercises below.

- Stare straight ahead of you (or at the ceiling if you are lying down).
- Take a deep breath in for a count of 4 to 8.
- Hold it for a count of 1.
- Exhale for a count of 4 to 8.
- Repeat these breaths three or five times.

Proceed to "One-Step Guided Imagery" or "Three-Step Guided Imagery."

One-Step Guided Imagery

Continue the deep breathing exercise. Have participants visualize their bodies becoming more vital and their minds more alert with each deep breath: "As you breathe in, feel your body becoming more energized and your mind more alert. As you breathe out, release all tension." Repeat, substituting your own words for *energized* and *alert*.

Three-Step Guided Imagery

1. Relaxation Imagery. Begin to focus on your toes. They are very relaxed. Take this relaxed feeling of warmth in the toes and imagine the relaxation moving up your legs, knees, and thighs. You are beginning to feel relaxed all over your body. Imagine this relaxation moving through your buttocks, lower abdomen, and lower back. This relaxation is slowly moving up your spine, vertebra by vertebra. This warmth is relaxing your abdomen, upper back, chest, neck, and face.

Now take this warmth, and feel it in your shoulders, down your arms, through your elbows, wrists, hands, and fingers. The warmth is now moving through your neck and up to your face. Relax your jaw and cheek muscles. Imagine the warmth circling around each eye. Relax your forehead and scalp. Your body feels relaxed and warm from your toes to your head. Sit with this warm feeling throughout your body, and feel relaxed and at peace.

2. Beach Get-away Imagery. Now imagine that you are walking on the beach. It is a sunny day and you can feel the warmth of the sun on your back. A gentle ocean breeze touches your face and leaves the taste of salt water on your lips. You lie down on a towel and begin to touch the warm sand with your toes. You feel warm and comfortable. The rhythmic sound of the waves carries your worries away. You are feeling relaxed and at peace with the world. Let this image and feeling evolve and change. Never force the image; merely go where your relaxed mind takes you.

3. Conclusion When you are ready, slowly wiggle your toes and fingers. Slowly open your eyes. Take a deep relaxing breath, and continue with your day, keeping in mind this beautiful and warm experience.

Deep-Breathing Exercise and *Three-Step Guided Imagery* were adapted from M.E. Copeland, 1994. *The depression workbook*. Oakland, CA: New Harbinger.

FIGURE 7.1 Guided imagery with deep-breathing exercise.

- The variations and progression options in the section "Illustrated Stretching Instruction" at the end of this chapter include the basic standing stretching exercises.
- If a participant has difficulty with a standing stretch, he or she can do the corresponding seated stretch.

Familiarize yourself and your participants with the body parts and major muscles targeted by each stretching exercise (see table 7.4). This information can help your participants focus on the body part or major muscles they are stretching. You may make a copy of table 7.4 to refer to during class.

TABLE 7.4 | Basic Standing Stretching Exercises

Target body parts and major muscles	Standing upper-body stretches	Page
Neck (neck extensors)	7.1 Standing Chin to Chest	162
Neck (neck rotators and extensors)	7.2 Standing Chin to Shoulder	163
Chest (pectoralis major) Shoulders (deltoids) Front upper arms (biceps)	[m,s]7.3 Standing Swan	163
Back (latissimus dorsi) Shoulders (deltoids)	7.4 Standing Half Hug	164
Back upper arms (triceps) Back (latissimus dorsi)	[m,s]7.5 Standing Zipper Stretch	165
Side of torso (abdominals)	7.6 Standing Side Bends	166
Torso (abdominals, spinal erectors)	[m,s]7.7 Standing Spinal Twist	167
Target body parts and major muscles	**Standing lower-body stretches**	**Page**
Back of thighs (hamstrings) Back (spinal erectors)	[m,s]7.8 Standing Tib Touches	169
Front thighs (quadriceps) Hips (hip flexors) Shins (tibialis anterior)	[s]7.9 Standing Quad Stretch (challenger)	170
Inner thighs (hip adductors)	[s]7.10 Standing Half-Splits	172
Outer hips and thighs (hip abductors)	[s]7.11 Standing Outer-Thigh Stretch	173
Calves (gastrocnemius, soleus)	[m,s]7.12 Standing Calf Stretch	175

The five exercises preceded by an *m* are recommended for a minimal stretching routine. The eight exercises preceded by an *s* are recommended for a short stretching routine.

From *Exercise for Frail Elders* by E. Best-Martini and K. A. Botenhagen-DiGenova, 2003, Champaign, IL: Human Kinetics.

Variations and Progression

The section "Illustrated Stretching Instruction" at the end of the chapter gives variations and progression options for each basic seated stretching exercise. You can introduce one or more of these variations after your participants have learned the basic seated exercises. Some classes, for example, a large class without an assistant in a long-term care setting, may be limited in how far they can progress, but varying the basic seated exercises can still add to the enjoyment of your class. Other classes may be able to do all standing stretches.

The most important progression option is the standing exercises. Standing exercises offer participants the greatest benefits in functional mobility and increased independence. Each basic seated exercise has a standing alternative. The benefits of the standing variations and when the seated version is preferred are discussed in chapter 8.

There are countless ways of varying and progressing an exercise program. For example, since the pectoralis major muscle (chest) is prone to tightness, it can be beneficial to do the Seated Swan (exercise 7.3) and a variation, such as the Seated Swan combined with extending the wrist. For many other ideas for varying and progressing your class, see chapter 8.

SUMMARY

This chapter gives simple guidelines, safety precautions, and teaching instructions for leading cool-down exercises. Always end your exercise class with a cool-down of 10 minutes at a minimum to ease the transition from exercise to rest and to enhance flexibility and relaxation.

For beneficial results, stretch all major muscle groups of the body two to seven days per week, repeating each stretch three to five times for 10 to 30 seconds per static stretch. Static (held or sustained) stretching is a safe, effective, and convenient method of stretching. It is common for elderly people, especially those who have been inactive, to have diminished flexibility that reduces their ability to perform daily activities independently. Participants who regularly stretch will have greater freedom of movement and increase their ability to perform activities of daily living.

ILLUSTRATED STRETCHING INSTRUCTION

Exercises 7.1 to 7.7 are upper-body stretching exercises, and exercises 7.8 to 7.12 are lower-body stretching exercises. The "Exercise and Safety Tips" and "Variations and Progression Options" apply to both seated and standing exercises unless otherwise specified. The standing exercises and other variations and progression options that need further explanation are accompanied by a photograph and description.

UPPER-BODY STRETCHING EXERCISES	EXERCISE 7.1

SEATED CHIN TO CHEST

Target Muscles   Neck (neck extensors)

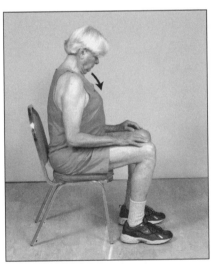

A

STRETCH POSITION

1. Good seated posture.*
2. Lower chin toward chest.
3. Feel stretch in back of neck.
4. Hold for less than 5 seconds.

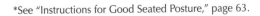
Exercise and Safety Tips

- Slowly lower the head and slowly lift it back to the starting position. Prevent the risk of neck injury by not lowering the head backward.
- Those without balance problems can eventually add the interlaced-fingers variation while standing.

*See "Instructions for Good Seated Posture," page 63.

(continued)

(continued)

Variations and Progression Options

- Combine Chin to Chest with interlaced fingers, pressing downward behind the back.
- Standing Chin to Chest.

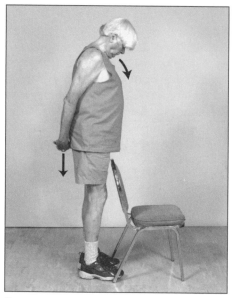

B

STANDING CHIN TO CHEST PLUS INTERLACED FINGERS

1. Good standing posture.
2. Hands behind back.
3. Interlace fingers.
4. Press downward.
5. Lower chin toward chest.
6. Feel stretch in back of neck.
7. Hold for less than 5 seconds.

EXERCISE 7.2	UPPER-BODY STRETCHING EXERCISES

SEATED CHIN TO SHOULDER

Target Muscles   Neck (neck rotators and extensors)

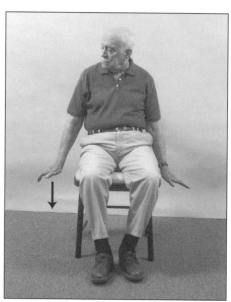

A

STRETCH POSITION

1. Good seated posture.*
2. Arms by sides.
3. Press palms downward.
4. Turn chin toward shoulder.
5. Feel stretch on side of neck.
6. Hold for less than 5 seconds.
7. Repeat toward other side.

*See "Instructions for Good Seated Posture," page 63.

Exercise and Safety Tips

- If chair arms are in the way when pressing palms downward, sitting on hands can also help keep the shoulders down.
- Those without balance problems can eventually add the interlaced-fingers variation while standing.

Variations and Progression Options

- Combine Chin to Shoulder with interlaced fingers, pressing downward behind the back.
- Standing Chin to Shoulder.

UPPER-BODY STRETCHING EXERCISES	EXERCISE 7.3

SEATED SWAN

Target Muscles Chest (pectoralis major), shoulders (deltoids), front upper arms (biceps)

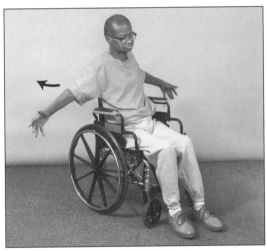

A

STRETCH POSITION

1. Good seated posture.*
2. Extend arms backward.
3. Palms face forward.
4. Keep shoulders down.
5. Feel stretch in chest and arms.
6. Hold for 10 to 30 seconds.

Exercise and Safety Tips

- Do not hyperextend (lock) the elbows.

Variations and Progression Options

- Palms facing upward or downward.
- Combine the Swan stretch with extending the wrist (fingers toward back of the arm) to stretch the front forearms (forearm flexors).
- Combine the Swan stretch with flexing the wrist (fingers toward front of the arm) to stretch the back of the forearms (forearm extensors).
- Standing Swan.
- Props: Hold a necktie, soft rope or towel between hands to enhance the Swan stretch.

*See "Instructions for Good Seated Posture," page 63.

SEATED HALF HUG

Target Muscles   Back (latissimus dorsi), shoulders (deltoids)

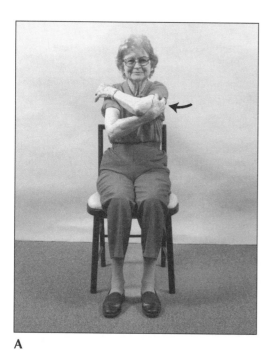

A

STRETCH POSITION

1. Good seated posture.*
2. Place fingertips on top of opposite shoulder.
3. Place other hand above elbow of opposite arm.
4. Push arm across chest.
5. Feel stretch in back and shoulder.
6. Hold for 10 to 30 seconds.
7. Repeat with the other arm.

Exercise and Safety Tips

- Keep shoulders down.

Variations and Progression Options

- Do Shoulder Shrugs (exercise 4.17 in chapter 4) or Shoulder Rotation (exercise 4.15 in chapter 4) after stretching each side.
- Standing Half Hug.

*See "Instructions for Good Seated Posture," page 63.

SEATED ZIPPER STRETCH

Target Muscles Back of upper arms (triceps), back (latissimus dorsi)

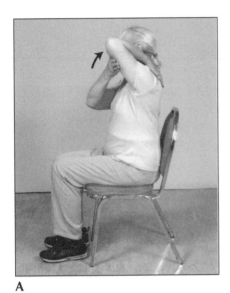

A

STRETCH POSITION

1. Good seated posture.*
2. Place fingertips on top of shoulder on same side, elbow up and pointing toward the front.
3. Place other hand on back of opposite upper arm.
4. Gently push arm backward.
5. Feel stretch in back of arm.
6. Hold for 10 to 30 seconds.
7. Repeat on other side.

Exercise and Safety Tips
- Do not overarch the back.
- Maintain a neutral spine throughout the stretch.

Variations and Progression Options
- Gently shake out arms after stretching on each side.
- Standing Zipper Stretch.
- Prop: Try Zipper Stretch using a towel, belt, or necktie.

STANDING ZIPPER STRETCH WITH PROP

1. Good standing posture.
2. Dangle prop over shoulder, behind back.
3. With other hand, grasp prop behind back.
4. Gently move the hands closer together along prop.
5. Feel stretch along back of arm and shoulder.
6. Hold for 10 to 30 seconds.
7. Repeat on other side.

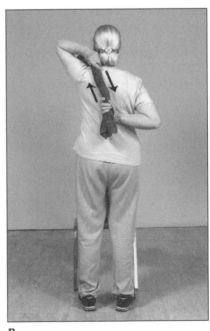

B

*See "Instructions for Good Seated Posture," page 63.

SEATED SIDE BENDS

Target Muscles Side of torso (abdominals)

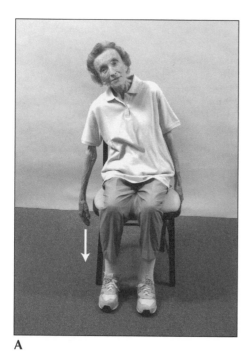

A

STRETCH POSITION

1. Good seated posture.*
2. Hold on to side of chair with one hand.
3. Other hand reaches toward floor.
4. Feel stretch along side.
5. Hold for 10 to 30 seconds.
6. Repeat on other side.

Exercise and Safety Tips

- Hold on to the arm or seat of the chair for support during Seated Side Bends.
- Do not bend the neck. Keep neck in a neutral position.

Variations and Progression Options

- Reach with one straight arm overhead and sideward, then repeat on the other side.
- Interlace fingers and reach straight arms overhead and sideward, then repeat on the other side.
- Gently shake out arms between stretches, especially when reaching overhead.
- Standing Side Bends.

*See "Instructions for Good Seated Posture," page 63.

SEATED SPINAL TWIST

Target Muscles   Torso (abdominals, spinal erectors)

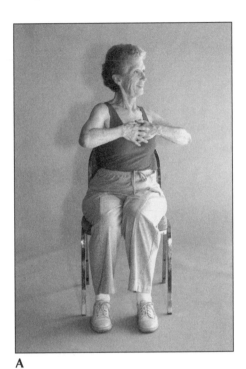

A

STRETCH POSITION
1. Good seated posture.*
2. Place palms on chest.
3. One hand on top of the other.
4. Elbows out.
5. Twist torso.
6. Feel stretch in front and back torso.
7. Hold for 10 to 30 seconds.
8. Repeat on other side.

Exercise and Safety Tips
- Do not twist the neck. Move the head, neck, and shoulders as a unit.
- Keep shoulders down.
- Modification: Lower elbows if shoulders get tired.

Variations and Progression Options
- Gently shake out the arms after stretching each side.
- Straight arms.
- Combine the Spinal Twist with lifting upward and visualizing getting taller with each exhalation.
- Standing Spinal Twist.

*See "Instructions for Good Seated Posture," page 63.

SEATED TIB TOUCHES (TIB FOR TIBIA OR SHIN BONE)

Target Muscles Back of thighs (hamstrings), back (spinal erectors)

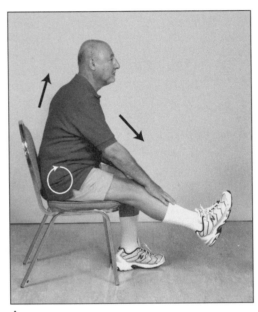

A

STRETCH POSITION
1. Good seated posture.*
2. Place palms on thighs.
3. Straighten one leg.
4. Slide hand down straight leg.
5. Bend forward at the hips.
6. Feel stretch in back of thigh.
7. Hold for 10 to 30 seconds.
8. Repeat with the other leg.

Exercise and Safety Tips
- Rest one palm on a thigh when leaning forward from the hips.
- Move head, neck, and spine as one unit. Do not hang head.
- Maintain a neutral spine (long and lifted) throughout the stretch.

Variations and Progression Options
- Combine Seated Tib Touches with a Calf Stretch (exercise 7.12).
- Prop: When seated, use a towel, strong resistance band, belt, or necktie around the ball of the foot for a calf stretch.
- Prop: Use a low stool to prop the foot up with Seated Tib Touches.
- Interlace fingers under outstretched leg.
- Standing Tib Touches.

*See "Instructions for Good Seated Posture," page 63.

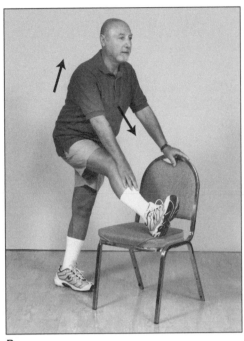

B

STANDING TIB TOUCHES

1. Good standing posture.
2. Place hand on chair back.
3. Place opposite heel on chair.
4. Slide free hand down straight leg.
5. Bend forward at the hips.
6. Feel stretch in back of thigh.
7. Hold for 10 to 30 seconds.
8. Repeat with the other leg.

LOWER-BODY STRETCHING EXERCISES	EXERCISE 7.9

SEATED QUAD STRETCH

Target Muscles   Front thighs (quadriceps), shins (tibialis anterior)

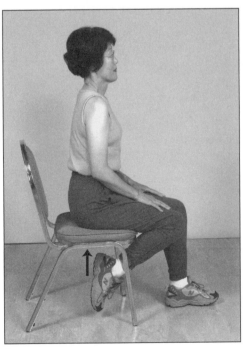

A

STRETCH POSITION

1. Good seated posture.*
2. Place palms on thighs.
3. Place front of toes on floor under chair (toe pointed).
4. Raise heel toward chair seat.
5. Feel stretch in front thigh and shin.
6. Hold for 10 to 30 seconds.
7. Repeat with the other leg.

*See "Instructions for Good Seated Posture," page 63.

(continued)

(continued)

Exercise and Safety Tips

- Modification: If there are bars between the front legs of the chairs, instruct participants to move forward 4 to 6 inches (10–15 centimeters) in their seats, if they can do so safely. Instruct them to hold on to the sides or arms of their chairs when sitting forward in the chair.
- There are several ways to hold up the calf in the Standing Quad Stretch: A participant can put his or her fingers in the top of the shoe or in the loop if the shoe has one; a less flexible person can hold on to the pants leg.
- Avoid leaning forward during the Standing Quad Stretch.
- Avoid locking the knee of the standing leg.

Variations and Progression Options

- Modification: Rest shin on chair seat in the Standing Quad Stretch instead of holding foot in hand. Focus on rotating the pelvis backward and point the toe to facilitate stretching the front thigh and shin, respectively.
- Standing Quad Stretch (challenger).

STANDING QUAD STRETCH (CHALLENGER)

1. Good standing posture.
2. Place hand on chair back.
3. Bend opposite knee (heel toward buttock).
4. With free hand, hold calf up (as directed in Exercise and Safety Tips).
5. Gently pull thigh and foot backward.
6. Feel stretch in front thigh and shin.
7. Hold for 10 to 30 seconds.
8. Repeat with the other leg.

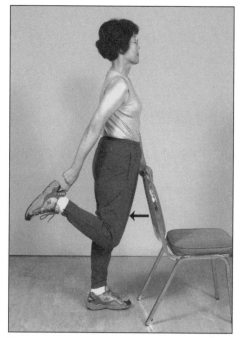

B

SEATED SPLITS

Target Muscles   Inner thighs (hip adductors)

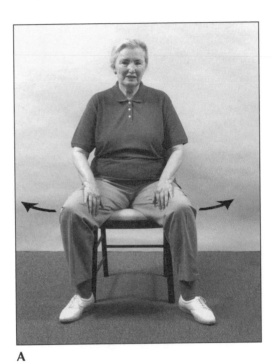

A

STRETCH POSITION

1. Good seated posture.*
2. Place palms on inner thighs.
3. Slide both feet outward.
4. Feel stretch in inner thighs.
5. Hold for 10 to 30 seconds.

Exercise and Safety Tips

- Keep each foot directly below each knee while doing Seated Splits.
- Press inner thighs outward gently to enhance the adductor stretch.
- Modification: If chairs with arms are used, tell participants to scoot forward in their chairs if they are comfortable doing so. Instruct them to hold on to the sides or arms of their chairs when sitting forward in the chair.

Variations and Progression Options

- Combine Seated Splits with a shoulder stretch by grasping under the thighs and bending elbows until shoulder stretch is felt.
- Standing Half-Splits.

*See "Instructions for Good Seated Posture," page 63.

(continued)

(continued)

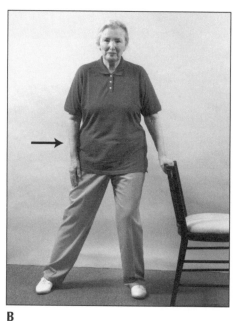

B

STANDING HALF-SPLITS

1. Good standing posture.
2. Place hands on chair back.
3. Move one foot sideward 1.5 to 2 feet (46–61 centimeters).
4. Slightly bend knee of other leg.
5. Lean into that leg.
6. Feel stretch in inner thigh of straight leg.
7. Hold for 10 to 30 seconds.
8. Repeat with the other leg.

EXERCISE 7.11	LOWER-BODY STRETCHING EXERCISES

SEATED OUTER-THIGH STRETCH

Target Muscles   Outer hips and thighs (hip abductors)

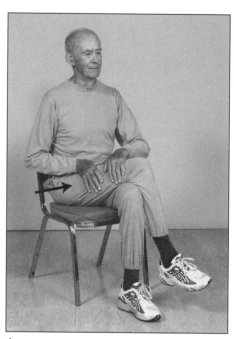

A

STRETCH POSITION

1. Good seated posture.*
2. Cross leg at knees.
3. Place palms on outer thigh.
4. Feel stretch in outer hip and thigh.
5. Hold for 10 to 30 seconds.
6. Repeat with the other leg.

*See "Instructions for Good Seated Posture," page 63.

Exercise and Safety Tips

- Anyone with peripheral vascular disease should avoid the seated crossed-leg position. Substitute the Standing Outer-Thigh Stretch if it can be done safely.
- When seated, gently pull the outer thigh inward (bring knee toward opposite shoulder).
- Avoid locking the knee of the standing leg.

Variations and Progression Options

- Gently twist the torso (not neck) toward the crossed leg while pulling the outer thigh inward.
- Standing Outer-Thigh Stretch.

STANDING OUTER-THIGH STRETCH

1. Good standing posture.
2. Place hand on chair back.
3. Cross one leg in front of the other.
4. Lean into the hip of the back leg.
5. Feel stretch in back leg's outer hip and thigh.
6. Hold for 10 to 30 seconds.
7. Repeat with the other leg.

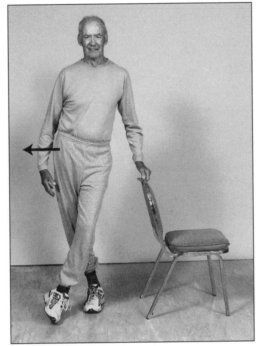

B

SEATED CALF STRETCH

Target Muscles   Calves (gastrocnemius, soleus)

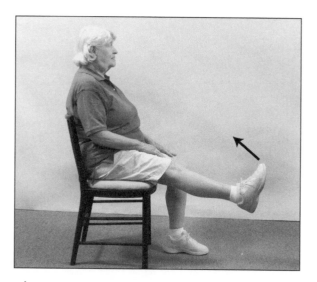

A

STRETCH POSITION
1. Good seated posture.*
2. Place palms on thighs.
3. Straighten one leg.
4. Dorsiflex ankle of straightened leg (toes toward nose).
5. Feel stretch in back of calf.
6. Hold for 10 to 30 seconds.
7. Repeat with the other leg.

Exercise and Safety Tips
- Keep the leg being stretched straight: knee soft, not locked.
- Perform the Standing Calf Stretch with the foot straight ahead of the calf that is being stretched.
- Keep the knee above the ankle of the forward standing leg.

Variations and Progression Options
- Prop: For the Seated Calf Stretch use a towel, strong resistance band, belt, or necktie around the ball of the foot to aid the calf stretch. This is easier when a stool is placed under the foot.
- Participants who are comfortable sitting forward in the chair can try the Seated Calf Stretch with the heel of the calf that is being stretched on the floor. Try using a prop (see previous bulleted point) to enhance this stretch.
- Standing Calf Stretch.

*See "Instructions for Good Seated Posture," page 63.

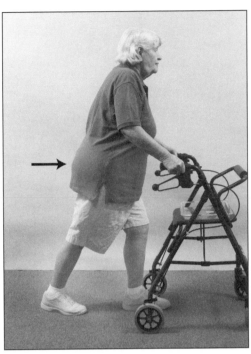

B

STANDING CALF STRETCH

1. Good standing posture.
2. Place hands on chair back.
3. Move one foot backward 1.5 to 2 feet (46–61 centimeters).
4. Toes point forward.
5. Slightly bend knee of forward leg.
6. Lean into that leg.
7. Feel stretch in calf of straight leg.
8. Hold for 10 to 30 seconds.
9. Repeat with the other leg.

CHAPTER 8

Putting Your Exercise Program Together

In this chapter you will discover how to implement a program that uses the warm-up, aerobic, resistance, and cool-down exercises from chapters 4 through 7. You will learn how to design, schedule, modify, progress (make progressively more challenging) or maintain, and monitor a smart fitness program for frail elders and adults with special needs.

Designing Your Exercise Program

There are many options for designing your exercise program, such as these:

- Leading one or more exercise components—warm-ups, aerobics, resistance training, and cool-down exercises—in one class.
- A comprehensive fitness class and program
- Leading just seated exercises, just standing exercises, or seated and standing exercises at the same time
- Leading just upper-body exercises, just lower-body ones, or both upper- and lower-body exercises
- Using exercise videotapes

Always consider the special needs of your participants when designing your exercise program.

Exercise Components

You can combine the exercise components in a variety of ways. Table 8.1 shows seven different ways, from a beginner-level class to a comprehensive fitness class. If you are starting an exercise class, we recommend the easiest-level class. Slowly progress toward the comprehensive fitness class.

All classes in table 8.1 include

- a warm-up session (which emphasizes joint ROM exercises but also includes posture, breathing, and stretching exercises),
- a relaxation component, at least deep breathing,
- an educational component, if only a quote (see "Focus on Education" and table 3.1 in chapter 3), and
- water breaks to prevent dehydration.

The boldface Xs indicate the focus of each class:

Level 1 focuses on relaxation exercises.

Level 2 focuses on warm-up ROM exercises. (Both levels 1 and 2 have the objective of motivating people to come back for more exercise and can include a discussion on a fitness-related topic with refreshments.)

Level 3 focuses on stretching.

Level 4 focuses on aerobics.

TABLE 8.1 EXERCISE PROGRAM OPTIONS

Exercise program components	Class level[a]						
	1	2	3	4	5	6	7
Warm-up ROM exercises	x	**X**	x	x	x	x	x
Aerobics				**X**		x	x
Resistance and balance exercises					**X**	**X**	x
Cool-down stretching			**X**	x	x	x	x
Cool-down relaxation exercises	**X**	x	x	x	x	x	x
Education	x	x	x	x	x	x	x
Healthy snacks	x	x					
Water breaks	x	x	x	x	x	x	x

[a]Classes progress from the easiest level (1) to a comprehensive fitness class (7). The boldface **X**s indicate the component that is emphasized in that class.

Level 5 focuses on resistance training and does not include aerobics.

Level 6 focuses on resistance training and includes aerobics.

Level 7 is a comprehensive fitness class that includes a warm-up, aerobics, resistance and balance exercises, and cool-down stretching and relaxation exercises.

Introduce only one new exercise component at a time. You do not have to teach all of the exercises in a component on the same day you introduce it. For example, you can start with four resistance exercises the first week, then add one new exercise each week for the following eight weeks. Initially, do more warm-up ROM exercises. As you increase the resistance exercises, cut back on the ROM component (but always warm up for at least 10 minutes). This easy-going approach to introducing new exercises is helpful for reinforcing good exercise technique and preventing overtraining.

Safety Tip

Introduce only one new exercise component—warm-up, aerobics, resistance training, or cool-down—at a time.

COMPREHENSIVE FITNESS PROGRAM

A *comprehensive* fitness class that includes a warm-up, aerobics, resistance and balance exercises, and a cool-down in *one class* is not necessarily a goal of an exercise program. But this format can be ideal for groups that meet only three or fewer times per week. Gradually build up to an hour of exercise, which a comprehensive fitness class requires.

Table 8.2 shows a sample weekly schedule for a comprehensive fitness program that meets four to five days per week. Notice the way that the exercise components are spread throughout the week. Aerobic and resistance training are offered the minimally recommended times per week (American College of Sports Medicine 1998b, 975). A comprehensive fitness class is offered once a week on Monday. Monday, the most strenuous day, is preceded by one or two days off and followed by an optional light workout. To prevent overtraining, avoid having strenuous workouts two days in a row. If the same group of people meet five times per week, one workout (Tuesday's, in this example) should be lighter, such as ROM or stretching and relaxation exercises only.

SEATED AND STANDING EXERCISES

You can teach the seated or standing versions of warm-up, aerobic, resistance, and stretching exercises. In this section you will find out:

- When a participant is ready for standing exercises
- The benefits of standing exercises
- When seated exercises are preferred over standing ones

TABLE 8.2 WEEKLY SCHEDULE FOR A COMPREHENSIVE FITNESS PROGRAM					
Fitness class components	Monday	Tuesday (optional)	Wednesday	Thursday	Friday or Saturday
Warm-up[a]	X	X	X	X	X
Aerobics	X		X		X
Resistance training	X[b]			X	
Cool-down	X	X	X	X	X

Classes are scheduled four to five days per week.

[a]The warm-up focuses on ROM exercises but also includes posture and breathing exercises and light stretches.

[b]You can move resistance training to Tuesdays if participants cannot tolerate a comprehensive fitness class.

When Is a Participant Ready for Standing Exercises?
When *all* the following criteria are true, a participant can perform standing exercises:

- The participant has become proficient with the basic seated exercises.
- The participant has no balance problems—or minor balance problems (only exercises that leave at least one hand free to hold on to a chair or other sturdy support are indicated), or major balance problems but has an experienced spotter for one-on-one facilitation. (Upper-body resistance exercises should still be done while the participant is seated when weights are used in both hands.)
- The participant has received medical clearance for standing exercises.
- The participant is not feeling fatigued.

What Are the Benefits of Standing Exercises?
There are remarkable benefits to standing exercises, so long as safety is not jeopardized. Some exercises are more effective or easier standing than seated, especially exercises for which the chair gets in the way. Other benefits of standing exercises include

- improved balance, particularly static standing balance,
- improved ability to perform daily activities that require standing,
- improved bone density and reduced risk of falls and bone fractures, and
- added exercise variety to your exercise program.

When Are Seated Exercises Preferred Over Standing?
Here are some guidelines for you to determine when a participant is better off doing seated exercises:

- When a participant fails to meet any of the previously discussed criteria for determining whether he or she is ready for standing exercises.
- When performing upper-body exercises that use both arms, particularly resistance exercises that require weights in both hands and thus preclude grasping a steady object for support if the participant loses his or her balance.
- When you want to save time by doing upper-body exercises on both sides simultaneously rather than one side at a time.
- When the participant no longer feels steady and balanced.
- When a participant can successfully and safely participate only in chair-seated exercise. For example, for those with Parkinson's disease, an all-seated exercise program is often the only safe option.

UPPER- AND LOWER-BODY EXERCISES

The exercises in chapters 4, 5, 6, and 7 are divided into upper- and lower-body exercises. You can teach upper- and lower-body exercises together or separately, except aerobic exercises (discussed a bit later). For example, if you start with the upper-body exercises, after your class is doing well with them, you may add on the lower-body exercises. Add them at a comfortable pace, even if just one exercise per class; a basic beginning fitness class for frail elders and adults with special needs can cover warm-up exercises during the first two or more weeks of class—the first class may include only upper-body exercises. Add the lower-body exercises over the next few classes.

With aerobic exercise, the lower- and upper-body movements go together. However, it is easier to learn the moves if the lower-body movements are taught first, then upper-body movements are added on. The lower-body movements, the foundation of aerobics, use large muscle groups, which are needed to sufficiently elevate one's heart rate for improving cardiovascular endurance. Encourage your participants to go at their own pace with aerobics. For instance, remind them that they may just do lower-body exercise if they start getting tired. Or, if their lower body needs a rest, they may do just upper-body movements. Alternatively, they may do the upper- and lower-body movements at a slower pace than the class.

EXERCISE VIDEOTAPES

Another option for your exercise class is to use an exercise videotape. Table 8.3 delineates the advantages and disadvantages of using exercise videos. Notice that some of the disadvantages can be turned into advantages. If you are interested in purchasing a videotape appropriate for frail elders and individuals with special needs, see the "Suggested Resources."

Consider videotaping your class. In your absence, a qualified leader (one who is trained in exercise supervision, knows the conditions and special needs of your participants, and understands all the safety guidelines) can pop in the video and supervise your class as they follow your lead.

SCHEDULING YOUR EXERCISE CLASSES

Schedule your exercise program so that your participants receive the greatest benefits. The following sections present general guidelines for the frequency and duration of your classes. Focus on safety: Increase either frequency or duration one at a time. Never increase both simultaneously, and increase them slowly.

CLASS FREQUENCY AND DURATION

A fitness class at least three times per week is optimal. Spread the classes throughout the week to give participants a longer recovery time between classes, which helps to prevent injuries. For example, meeting Monday, Wednesday, and Friday is preferable to Monday, Tuesday, and Wednesday. The sample schedule in table 8.2 is based on the American College of Sports Medicine's (1998b, 975) recommendations for frequency and duration.

Recommended Frequencies

Resistance training	Two to three times per week on nonconsecutive days
Aerobic training	Three to five days per week
Stretching	Two to three times per week minimum

TABLE 8.3 EXERCISE VIDEOTAPES

Advantages	Disadvantages
You can videotape your own class to be played in your absence.	Few good-quality videotapes are available for older adults and those with special needs.
Exposure to a variety of teaching styles can provide new insights.	Videotapes can be less motivational than a live instructor.
A less highly trained fitness leader can more easily supervise participants while they are following a videotape.	The class still needs to be carefully supervised while following an exercise videotape.
Instructor will have more time to modify an exercise for participants when needed during class.	Instructor may not pay as close attention to participants as when he or she is leading in front of the class. For example, those with visual or auditory deficits may not get needed special cues.
Videotapes can make it possible to offer classes more times per week and provide a more diverse exercise curriculum.	Participants may be less likely to come to class.

TABLE 8.4   FOUR EXAMPLES OF 45- TO 60-MINUTE EXERCISE CLASSES

A model warm-up–only class		A model resistance-training class	
Opening	5 minutes	Opening	5 minutes
Posture exercise	2 minutes	Warm-up	10 minutes
Breathing exercise	3 minutes	Resistance exercises	15–30 minutes
ROM exercises	20–25 minutes	Cool-down	10 minutes
Cool-down	10–20 minutes	Closing	5 minutes
Closing (e.g., cleaning weights)	5 minutes		45–60 minutes
	45–60 minutes		
A model aerobics class		**A model stretching and relaxation class**	
Opening	5 minutes	Opening	5 minutes
Warm-up	10 minutes	Warm-up	10 minutes
Aerobic exercises	15–30 minutes[a]	Stretching exercises	20–30 minutes
Cool-down	10 minutes	Relaxation exercises	5–10 minutes
Closing	5 minutes	Closing	5 minutes
	45–60 minutes		45–60 minutes

Times are approximate.

[a]Aerobics may be better tolerated if divided into short bouts (e.g., two to three 10-minute sessions) interspersed with low-level leg movement, such as ROM exercises.

A 1-hour exercise class is a good goal. Participants tend to drop out of programs that last longer than 1 hour per session (Balady et al. 2000, 160). Table 8.4 shows four examples of classes lasting 45 to 60 minutes. Each class focuses on a different exercise component: warm-up, aerobics, resistance training, or cool-down. Table 8.5 puts all the exercise components together into a model comprehensive fitness class that lasts 60 to 70 minutes. Each model class dedicates 5 minutes to opening and 5 minutes to closing the class. Chapter 3 gives helpful tips for opening and closing your exercise class.

Schedule a set amount of time, such as 45 to 60 minutes, for your exercise class. You can initially do fewer exercises and offer other activities, such as an educational or motivational lecture and discussion and healthy refreshments at the end. Educating people about the benefits of exercise can increase exercise adherence (see "Focus on Education" and table 3.1 in chapter 3). Refreshments are an extrinsic motivator for people who are resistant to exercise. Healthy snacks at the end of class are also rewarding and can make your class more popular among the less-motivated participants. On the other hand, some may prefer to leave when the exercises are over, so be flexible and leave the choice to each individual. Table 8.6 offers a possible schedule for you to start with. This sample class meets two or three days per week for 45 to 60 minutes and includes warm-up

TABLE 8.5   A MODEL COMPREHENSIVE FITNESS CLASS

Activity	Time (minutes)[a]
Opening	5
Warm-up	10
Aerobics	15–25[b]
Resistance training	15
Cool-down	10
Closing	5
Total class time	60–70

[a]Times are approximate.

[b]Including a 5-minute postaerobic cool-down before resistance training (see chapter 7).

exercises (posture, breathing, ROM, and stretching exercises), an educational component, and healthy refreshments. Work with the interests and abilities of your participants to gradually increase the exercise time and reduce the other activities. Also, be flexible with participants; for example, allow someone to attend one day per week initially if that is all he or she is ready for.

TABLE 8.6	WEEKLY SCHEDULE FOR A BEGINNER EXERCISE CLASS		
Exercise class components	**Monday**	**Wednesday (optional)**	**Friday**
Warm-up: posture, breathing, ROM, and stretching	15–20[a]	15–20	15–20
Education	15–20	15–20	15–20
Healthy refreshments	15–20	15–20	15–20

[a]Suggested times can be adjusted to meet the special needs of your participants.

DURATION OF THE EXERCISE COMPONENTS

Chapters 4 through 7 give comprehensive sets of warm-up, aerobic, resistance, and stretching exercises. The following sections give specific suggestions for shortening each exercise component or prolonging it to fill an entire class or to make it more challenging.

Bear in mind that the exercises take longer to lead in the initial learning phase. Practice the exercises before you start the class for a good sense of the timing, especially if you are a new fitness leader. The three-step instructional process in chapter 3 can help you demonstrate and describe each exercise clearly and systematically.

In general, you can shorten the comprehensive set of 24 warm-up exercises, 10 aerobic exercises, 12 resistance exercises, and 12 stretches by doing fewer exercises or fewer repetitions of each exercise.

Here are ways to extend a single warm-up, aerobic, resistance-training, or stretching component into an entire class. Initially, teaching all the basic exercises of an exercise component might fill an entire class. When your class is ready for a greater challenge, slowly introduce the following options:

- Repeat some of your participants' favorite exercises
- Repeat some or all of the basic exercises
- Add variations of some or all of the exercises
- Increase the number of repetitions of an exercise

Many factors influence the duration of an exercise component, such as

- class size,
- number of instructors and assistants,
- participants' need for assistance with equipment and individual exercises,
- instructor's and participants' experience with the exercises, and
- level of fitness of the participants.

Because of these variables, we recommend that you start with teaching just the warm-up exercises. Expand your exercise class from there, after you are familiar with your participants' needs and limitations and how long it takes to get through the warm-up.

DURATION OF WARM-UP

You may shorten or lengthen the duration of the warm-up to fit the special needs of your class, but you must warm up for *at least* 10 minutes before doing any other exercises. If you are leading more than one exercise component in a workout, you need to warm up only at the beginning of class, unless resistance training precedes aerobics (see chapter 4).

To shorten the warm-up, you can use one of these suggestions:

- Do as many of the 24 warm-up exercises as possible in an allotted time. In this case, you can do just the first couple of exercises for each joint in order to warm up the entire body.
- Concentrate on the major joints (hip, back, shoulder, knee, upper trunk, and neck regions).
- Do the upper-body exercises on both sides at the same time.
- Do fewer repetitions of each exercise (e.g., three or four instead of eight).

You can extend the warm-up exercise into an entire class by using one of these suggestions:

- Do the upper-body exercises on one side at a time (recommended when participants are learning the exercises).
- Repeat the warm-up exercises for a given joint, such as all the hip exercises

- Repeat a movement pattern at each joint, such as rotating all the joints.
- Increase the number of sets of a warm-up exercise.
- Intersperse more sets of an exercise throughout the warm-up.
- After participants have learned the basic exercises, combine an upper-body warm-up exercise with a lower-body warm-up exercise (e.g., Up-and-Down Leg March with Butterfly Wings). In general, upper- and lower-body stretching exercises should be done separately for safety and to help participants focus on the muscles being stretched.

Duration of Aerobics

You may shorten or lengthen the duration of the aerobics component to fit the special needs of your class. Remember to include at least a 10-minute warm-up before aerobics and a 10-minute cool-down after aerobics.

For a shorter aerobics segment, you can do as many of the 10 aerobic exercises as possible in an allotted time.

You can increase the aerobics component into an entire class by introducing new variations such as these:

- Integrate some or all of the additional arm movements.
- Create a pattern with 2 exercises (see "Other Training Techniques" in chapter 5).
- Create a combination with 2 or more patterns.

Duration of Resistance Training

You may shorten or lengthen the duration of the resistance-training component to fit the special needs of your class. Remember to include at least a 10-minute warm-up before resistance training and a 10-minute cool-down after resistance training.

For a shorter resistance segment, do just the eight exercises listed in table 8.7, the minimum number of recommended resistance exercises per workout. These eight resistance exercises strengthen the muscles that are notoriously weak for most older adults.

You can extend the duration of resistance exercises to fill an entire class by

- increasing the number of sets to two or three at most or
- increasing the number of repetitions to 15 maximum.

Duration of Stretching Exercises

You may shorten or lengthen the duration of the stretching component to fit the special needs of your class. Remember to warm up for at least 10 minutes before stretching.

If you are short on time toward the end of class, you can do one of the reduced sets of stretches listed in tables 4.3 and 4.4 in chapter 4. These shorter sets of stretching exercises include critical stretches for body parts that are notoriously tight for the majority of older adults.

TABLE 8.7 An Eight-Exercise Resistance-Training Component

Basic seated resistance exercises	Page	Basic standing resistance and balance exercises	Page
6.1 Seated Chest Press	135	6.1 Standing Chest Press	135
6.2 Seated Two-Arm Row	136	6.2 Standing Two-Arm Row	137
6.3 Seated Overhead Press	138	6.3 Standing Overhead Press	138
6.6 Modified Chair Stands (challenger)[a]	141	6.6 Chair Stands (challenger)[a]	142
6.7 Seated Hip Flexion	143	6.7 Standing Hip Flexion	143
6.8 Seated Hip Abduction and Adduction	144	6.8 Standing Hip Abduction and Adduction	145
6.11 Seated Toe Raises	149	6.11 Standing Toe Raises	149
6.12 Seated Heel Raises	150	6.12 Standing Heel Raises	150

[a]Add the challenger exercise after participants are comfortable with the other seven exercises.

You can extend the stretching exercises into an entire class by

- increasing the length of time that you hold the stretches up to 1 minute or
- repeating a stretch up to five times.

MODIFYING THE EXERCISES

Not all the basic seated and standing exercises are appropriate for all participants. Refer to participants' medical clearance forms to see whether the physician or physical therapist has made any special exercise recommendations. If you have tried the following suggestions but are still unable to modify an exercise so that a participant can perform it successfully, ask his or her medical professionals for recommendations for alternative exercises. If your class is large and you do not have an assistant, you may need to ask a participant to stay after class for further individual instruction.

When to Modify an Exercise
You might need to modify an exercise when a participant has one or more of the following:

- Problems performing an exercise
- Problems keeping up with the class
- Special needs
- Pain (also see table 2.1 and figure 2.1 in chapter 2)

How to Modify an Exercise
There are several ways to modify an exercise for a participant:

- **Decrease the workload.** Decrease the number of repetitions of the exercise, the number of sets, the amount of weight or resistance (for resistance exercises), or a combination of these.
- **Adjust the exercise technique.** If a participant is not using proper exercise technique, further verbal and visual cues may help. Sometimes gently leading a participant hand over hand (your hand over their hand) through a few repetitions of an exercise using proper exercise technique can help. Remember to ask permission before touching a participant.
- **Adjust the body position.** A participant may be performing the exercise in an awkward position or with poor posture. This can be a good time to remind the entire class about good posture.
- **Adjust the speed of the movement.** Have the participant decrease the speed of movement if

he or she is moving faster than you. Faster movements increase risk of injury. Allow participants to go slower than the pace of the class if that is more comfortable for him or her.
- **Consult the physician or physical therapist.** Always ask a participant to stop exercising if he or she experiences any pain. If the participant continues to feel pain after trying the suggested modifications, consult with his or her physician or physical therapist. Ask the physician or physical therapist to recommend another exercise.

Start with one modification to address the most obvious need. For example, if the participant is slouching, adjust the body position. If that modification is unsuccessful, try another. It can be helpful to refer to the "Specific Precautions for Those With Special Needs" sections in chapters 4 through 7.

PROGRESSING YOUR EXERCISE CLASS

Progression is not necessarily linear; your participants' abilities vary from day to day, and they may have to go back to an easier level if they have missed classes. Some participants need encouragement to progress in their workouts, while others need reminders not to push too hard. In this section, you will learn more about when and how to make your class progressively more challenging, including instructions for progressing each exercise component, challenger exercises, and variation and progression options. Remember our "K.I.S.S.S. principle"—keep your class simple, safe, and slowly progress:

• **Keep it simple.** We recommend that you start with only one component: an extended warm-up session of posture, breathing, gentle range-of-motion, and stretching exercises. This gives your participants a chance to feel successful before progressing to another exercise component (aerobics, resistance training, or cool-down exercises). Bear in mind that your class may be some participants' first experience with a fitness program as adults, and they may feel intimidated by too much information early on.

• **Keep it safe.** Introducing one exercise component at a time gives participants time to safely adjust to each exercise, and it allows you time to closely observe and get to know the group. As you learn the strengths and limitations of your participants, you can appropriately pace the progression of your class.

• **Progress slowly.** Slowly introduce new exercises. Gradually make your class more challenging. Because people start at different levels of fitness and progress at different rates, continually give participants permission to do the exercises at their own pace. For instance, if the aerobics pace is too fast for a participant, he or she can do one move for every two that you lead. Discourage competition among participants. Encourage participants to progress gradually in their workouts and, most important, to attend class regularly. Regular attendance is key to successful progression.

What are the signs that your participants are ready to progress?

• Their exercise technique is good.
• They have no signs of fatigue. In general, your participants should feel energized or only mildly fatigued at the end of class.
• When you ask them, "Are you ready for some new exercises?" they say, "Yes!"

If some are ready to progress while others are not, the ones who are not can take a water break during the new exercises. Encourage them to join in when they are ready.

The rate at which your class progresses and the levels that participants reach depend on several factors, such as

• physicians' or physical therapists' recommendations
• participants' goals, motivations, and abilities,
• your enthusiasm,
• the size of the class,
• the duration and frequency of the class, and
• the equipment available.

There are two general modes of progression. You should use only one mode at a time.

1. Adding a fitness component (warm-up, aerobics, resistance training, or stretching and relaxation exercises) to your class.
2. Adding to a fitness component of your class, as in these examples:
   • Add one or more new exercises per class, depending on the time available and how quickly participants learn new exercises.
   • Add the lower-body exercises after the upper-body exercises have been learned, or vice versa.

• You can add standing exercises for *ambulatory* (able to walk) participants after they have learned the seated exercises. If you are working one-on-one with a nonambulatory client who has physician approval for standing exercises, begin with one standing exercise and gradually increase the number of standing exercises performed. Your client should do the exercise seated when he or she becomes fatigued.

HOW TO PROGRESS THE FREQUENCY, INTENSITY, AND DURATION OF EACH EXERCISE COMPONENT

Gradually increase the frequency, intensity, and duration of each exercise component to meet the goals and needs of your class. In general, it is prudent to increase only one parameter (frequency, intensity, or duration) at a time. For example, if you increase the frequency by one session per week, postpone increasing the duration or intensity until participants have adapted to the extra day of exercise. Keep in mind that the exercise guidelines in chapters 4 through 7 give recommendations for progression.

CHALLENGER EXERCISES

The exercises labeled "challenger" in chapters 4 through 7 are exercises that many participants have difficulty learning in the beginning of a fitness class. Give your participants an opportunity to feel successful in your exercise class by introducing these more-challenging exercises after they are comfortable with the other basic exercises. Participants who attend class regularly will improve their physical fitness and be better able to perform the challengers. For example, the Seated Modified Chair Stands and regular Chair Stands are both challenger exercises that are easier after participants have increased their leg strength with the other seated lower-body resistance exercises. When your class is ready for something new, we recommend introducing the challenger exercises first, then the variations and progression options.

VARIATIONS AND PROGRESSION OPTIONS

Chapters 4 through 7 offer variations and progression options for each exercise component. The variations and progression options enable you to design a creative and progressive fitness program and adapt it to meet participants' needs.

MAINTAINING FITNESS RESULTS

An effective exercise program is dynamic, regularly changing to meet participants' needs. Even a program designed to maintain exercise at a current level is not static. If a participant gets ill, for instance, he or she should resume exercise at an easier level and slowly progress to his or her maintenance level. Whether progressing or maintaining their exercise, participants have day-to-day variations in their ability for physical activity.

Whether a participant is ready to stop progressing and start maintaining his or her exercise program depends on several factors, including his or her short- and long-term goals, motivation, physical and mental ability, the physician's or physical therapist's recommendations, and the equipment available. Reevaluate short-term and long-term goals before entering the maintenance stage (see "Goal Setting" in chapter 2).

Some participants in an exercise class may be maintaining their exercise levels, while others are progressing. In addition, some may be maintaining one component of exercise (e.g., resistance training) and progressing in another (e.g., aerobics training). Some participants cannot progress very far and thus reach the maintenance phase earlier than others. For example, it is not safe for those with dementia to lift more than a 1-pound (0.5-kilogram) free weight, which could injure them if dropped.

When participants are maintaining a current level of fitness, focus on varying their exercises. The variation options in chapters 4 through 7 make that easy.

MONITORING ATTENDANCE AND PROGRESS

A key to each individual's success in your exercise class is recording his or her attendance and progress. This can be a powerful motivator to keep them coming back to your class. Figure 3.3 (in chapter 3) shows a fun and effective way to record attendance. Design a chart to suit your class. You can write the time spent doing physical activity or use stickers as an engaging way to acknowledge attendance.

A log is particularly useful to keep track of resistance training. You may copy the Resistance Training Log in appendix K. A log helps a participant see progress achieved over weeks and months and encourages him or her to accomplish even more. When you have records about the weights everyone is using, workouts go more quickly and smoothly.

SUMMARY

One size does not fit all when teaching a fitness class to frail elders and adults with special needs. This chapter provided information about designing, scheduling, progressing, modifying, maintaining, and monitoring a personalized fitness program. Since most adults have special needs, if only a previous orthopedic injury, you are now equipped to work with all older adults. We wish you the best in guiding the individuals in your class toward better fitness for living a full and active life.

PHYSIOLOGICAL BENEFITS OF PHYSICAL ACTIVITY FOR OLDER PERSONS

IMMEDIATE BENEFITS

- **Glucose levels:** Physical activity helps regulate blood glucose levels.
- **Catecholamine activity:** Both adrenaline and noradrenaline levels are stimulated by physical activity.
- **Improved sleep:** Physical activity has been shown to enhance sleep quality and quantity in individuals of all ages.

LONG-TERM EFFECTS

- **Aerobic/cardiovascular endurance:** Substantial improvements in almost all aspects of cardiovascular functioning have been observed following appropriate physical training.

- **Resistive training/muscle strengthening:** Individuals of all ages can benefit from muscle-strengthening exercises. Resistance training can have a significant impact on the maintenance of independence in old age.
- **Flexibility:** Exercise that stimulates movement throughout the range of motion assists in the preservation and restoration of flexibility.
- **Balance/coordination:** Regular activity helps prevent or postpone the age-associated declines in balance and coordination that are a major risk factor for falls.
- **Velocity of movement:** Behavioral slowing is a characteristic of advancing age. Individuals who are regularly active can often postpone these age-related declines.

Appendix B

Psychological Benefits of Physical Activity for Older Persons

Immediate Benefits

- **Relaxation:** Appropriate physical activity enhances relaxation.
- **Reduces stress and anxiety:** There is evidence that regular physical activity can reduce stress and anxiety.
- **Enhanced mood state:** Numerous people report improvement in mood state following appropriate physical activity.

Long-Term Effects

- **General well-being:** Improvements in almost all aspects of psychological functioning have been observed following periods of extended physical activity.

- **Improved mental health:** Regular exercise can make an important contribution in the treatment of several mental illnesses, including depression and anxiety neurosis.
- **Cognitive improvements:** Regular physical activity may help postpone age-related declines in central nervous system processing speed and improve reaction time.
- **Motor control and performance:** Regular activity helps prevent or postpone the age-associated declines in both fine and gross motor performance.
- **Skills acquisition:** New skills can be learned and existing skills refined by all individuals regardless of age.

Reprinted from *The Heidelberg Guidelines for Promoting Physical Activity Among Older Persons* (WHO 1997). The WHO Guidelines have been placed in the public domain and can be freely copied and distributed. From *Exercise for Frail Elders* by E. Best-Martini and K. A. Botenhagen-DiGenova, 2003, Champaign, IL: Human Kinetics.

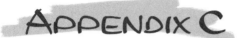

Statement of Medical Clearance for Exercise

Participant's name: _____

Address: _____

Date of birth: _____

Diagnosis: _____

Physician's name: _____

Address: _____

Telephone number: _____

❑ YES. My patient _____ has no current unstable medical problems that are a contraindication to participating in an exercise or resistance-training program. I approve of and support his or her participation in this progressive strength, balance, and flexibility-training exercise program.

Comments:

❑ NO. My patient _____ is not eligible to participate in the exercise program due to his or her current medical status.

Comments:

Please indicate any special recommendations or specific comments:

_____

_____

_____

_____

_____   _____
Physician's signature   Date

From *Exercise for Frail Elders* by E. Best-Martini and K. A. Botenhagen-DiGenova, 2003, Champaign, IL: Human Kinetics.

COVER LETTER TO PHYSICIAN

(For use with the medical clearance form in appendix C.)

_____ [Date]

Dear Dr. _____ ,

Your patient, _____ , is interested in participating in an exercise class, which

may include resistance training, at _____ [name of facility].
The goals of this program are to improve muscular strength, balance, and functional fitness in older adults.

We are enclosing a statement of medical clearance for exercise and request that you indicate your
patient's eligibility for this program. Please be sure to include any specific exercise recommendations or
adaptations to address your patient's needs.

If you have any questions regarding this exercise program or your patient's participation, please contact

me at _____ [phone number].

Sincerely,

_____ [Name]

_____ [Title]

Appendix E

Medical History and Risk Factor Questionnaire

Date: _____

Name: _____ Age: _____

Emergency contact and phone number:

_____

Medical history: Have you ever had, or do you currently have, any of the following?

❑ Abnormal EKG

❑ Anemia

❑ Arthritis

❑ Asthma

❑ Cancer

❑ Cardiac problems

❑ Chest pains

❑ Diabetes

❑ Emphysema

❑ Fainting

❑ High blood pressure

❑ High cholesterol

❑ Hypoglycemia

❑ Irregular heart beats

❑ Memory loss

❑ Osteoporosis

❑ Parkinson's disease

❑ Phlebitis

❑ Pulmonary disorder

❑ Shortness of breath

❑ Stroke (CVA)

❑ Injury to:

    ❑ shoulder

    ❑ wrist

    ❑ back

    ❑ hip

    ❑ knee

    ❑ other:

From *Exercise for Frail Elders* by E. Best-Martini and K. A. Botenhagen-DiGenova, 2003, Champaign, IL: Human Kinetics.

195

Do you take any medications? If so, please list all of them.

_____

_____

_____

_____

Are you experiencing any pain? ❏ NO ❏ YES   If yes, where is the pain felt?

_____

_____

Do you have any movement limitations? ❏ NO ❏ YES   If yes, please describe.

_____

_____

Are you currently receiving physical, occupational, or speech therapy? ❏ NO ❏ YES   If yes, what type and for what reason?

_____

_____

Do you consider yourself to be active, moderately active, slightly active, or sedentary (inactive)? (Circle one.)

Active   Moderately active   Slightly active   Sedentary (inactive)

Describe how often, how intensely (light, moderate, hard), and how long you exercise. What type of exercise?_____

_____

List one fitness goal that you would like to achieve:

_____

_____

Are there any physical movements that you would like to be able to do more easily (for example, scratching your back, picking something up off the floor)? If so, please list them.

_____

_____

Thanks for your time and information!

From *Exercise for Frail Elders* by E. Best-Martini and K. A. Botenhagen-DiGenova, 2003, Champaign, IL: Human Kinetics.

EXERCISE PROGRAM INFORMED CONSENT

The risks and benefits of this exercise program have been reviewed and explained to me. I understand and confirm that I will choose the level of activity that will not harm me. In consideration of my participation in this exercise program, I hereby release

_____ ,

[Name of facility]

its officers, employees, or agents from any liability for my personal injury or otherwise, arising out of or in any way connected to my participation in this exercise program.

Name: _____ Date: _____

Signature: _____

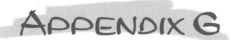

Physical Activity Readiness
Questionnaire – PAR-Q
(revised 1994)

PAR - Q & YOU

(A Questionnaire for People Aged 15 to 69)

Regular physical activity is fun and healthy, and increasingly more people are starting to become more active every day. Being more active is very safe for most people. However, some people should check with their doctor before they start becoming much more physically active.

If you are planning to become much more physically active than you are now, start by answering the seven questions in the box below. If you are between the ages of 15 and 69, the PAR-Q will tell you if you should check with your doctor before you start. If you are over 69 years of age, and you are not used to being very active, check with your doctor.

Common sense is your best guide when you answer these questions. Please read the questions carefully and answer each one honestly: check YES or NO.

YES	NO	
☐	☐	1. Has your doctor ever said that you have a heart condition <u>and</u> that you should only do physical activity recommended by a doctor?
☐	☐	2. Do you feel pain in your chest when you do physical activity?
☐	☐	3. In the past month, have you had chest pain when you were not doing physical activity?
☐	☐	4. Do you lose your balance because of dizziness or do you ever lose consciousness?
☐	☐	5. Do you have a bone or joint problem that could be made worse by a change in your physical activity?
☐	☐	6. Is your doctor currently prescribing drugs (for example, water pills) for your blood pressure or heart condition?
☐	☐	7. Do you know of <u>any other reason</u> why you should not do physical activity?

If you answered

YES to one or more questions

Talk with your doctor by phone or in person BEFORE you start becoming much more physically active or BEFORE you have a fitness appraisal. Tell your doctor about the PAR-Q and which questions you answered YES.

- You may be able to do any activity you want—as long as you start slowly and build up gradually. Or, you may need to restrict your activities to those which are safe for you. Talk with your doctor about the kinds of activities you wish to participate in and follow his/her advice.
- Find out which community programs are safe and helpful for you.

NO to all questions

If you answered NO honestly to all PAR-Q questions, you can be reasonably sure that you can:

- start becoming much more physically active—begin slowly and build up gradually. This is the safest and easiest way to go.
- take part in a fitness appraisal—this is an excellent way to determine your basic fitness so that you can plan the best way for you to live actively.

DELAY BECOMING MUCH MORE ACTIVE:

- if you are not feeling well because of a temporary illness such as a cold or a fever—wait until you feel better; or
- if you are or may be pregnant—talk to your doctor before you start becoming more active.

Please note: If your health changes so that you then answer YES to any of the above questions, tell your fitness or health professional. Ask whether you should change your physical activity plan.

<u>Informed Use of the PAR-Q:</u> The Canadian Society for Exercise Physiology, Health Canada, and their agents assume no liability for persons who undertake physical activity, and if in doubt after completing this questionnaire, consult your doctor prior to physical activity.

You are encouraged to copy the PAR-Q but only if you use the entire form

NOTE: If the PAR-Q is being given to a person before he or she participates in a physical activity program or a fitness appraisal, this section may be used for legal or administrative purposes.

I have read, understood and completed this questionnaire. Any questions I had were answered to my full satisfaction.

NAME _____

SIGNATURE _____ DATE _____

SIGNATURE OF PARENT _____ WITNESS _____
or GUARDIAN (for participants under the age of majority)

Reprinted from the 1994 revised version of the Physical Activity Readiness Questionnaire (PAR-Q and YOU). The PAR-Q and YOU is a copyrighted, pre-exercise screen, owned by the Canadian Society for Exercise Physiology. From *Exercise for Frail Elders* by E. Best-Martini and K. A. Botenhagen-DiGenova, 2003, Champaign, IL: Human Kinetics.

APPENDIX H
FITNESS GOAL MAP

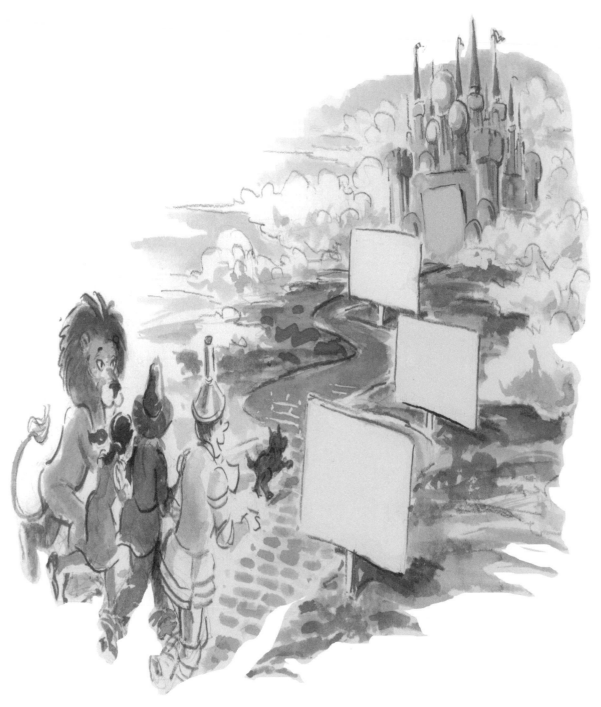

Adapted, by permission, from S.N. Blair, et al., 2001, *Active living everyday* (Champaign, IL: Human Kinetics), 55. From *Exercise for Frail Elders* by E. Best-Martini and K. A. Botenhagen-DiGenova, 2003, Champaign, IL: Human Kinetics.

EXERCISE EQUIPMENT

Type of equipment	Exercise component	Special needs/adaptations	How to use and other considerations
Ankle and wrist weights	Resistance training	Wrist weights are better than hand weights for beginner frail elders, adults with arthritis in their hands, and those with hemiparesis or hemiplegia from a stroke.	The weight is worn on the wrist and does not need to be held in the hand.
Balls, small rubber (5–10 inches, or 13–25 centimeters, in diameter)	Warm-ups Resistance training	Develop coordination, increase hand strength. Helpful before using dumbbells. Smaller balls can be held by those having contractures in their hands.	Start the warm-up with one ball per participant, to be used for hand exercises. Participants can also pass the balls around the circle.
Beanbags (large)	Warm-ups Resistance training Stretching	Improve body awareness, posture, and balance of all participants, especially those with stroke or neurological disorders resulting in loss of sensation. Good for proprioception (awareness of posture and changes of equilibrium during exercises).	Large beanbags, for sitting on the floor, are recommended only with physician or physical therapist approval.
Box lids	Warm-ups Resistance training Stretching	For individuals whose legs cannot touch the floor when seated.	Place in front of chair so that the participant can exercise with feet firmly planted.
Cans (food) of different sizes	Resistance training	Cans can be used instead of dumbbells	Use with caution if the participant has arthritis in the hands or cannot hold can firmly.
Dowels, wooden (2–4 feet, or 61–122 centimeters, long)	ROM Resistance training	The length depends on the ROM of participants.	Use a light dowel for ROM exercises.
Dumbbells (also called free weights or hand weights)	Resistance training	For those who have problems holding on to a dumbbell, weights with handles can be easier to hold (see ankle and wrist weights).	Cast-iron dumbbells are the least expensive type of free weights. They are commonly available in the United States in weights of 1, 2, 3, 5, 8, 10, 12, and 15 pounds (and more). Neoprene and vinyl-covered weights typically come in weights from 1 to 12 pounds in 1-pound increments, and each weight is a different color—a fun extrinsic motivator. However, they are significantly more expensive than cast-iron weights.

(continued)

(continued)

Type of equipment	Exercise component	Special needs/adaptations	How to use and other considerations
Handkerchiefs, scarves	Warm-ups Stretching	Good for visual stimulation	Good visual reminders to use full-ROM movements.
Microphone	Warm-ups Aerobics Resistance training Stretching	Hearing loss	A cordless microphone is ideal, as the fitness leader can move around and be heard clearly by all in the class.
Mirrors	Warm-ups Aerobics Resistance training Stretching	Participants who have had a stroke are often unaware of the affected side of their bodies. A mirror helps bring both sides together for them. Be aware that some participants with dementia do not feel comfortable with their reflection in a mirror.	A mirror on a wall or door mirror enables participants to watch their technique.
Newspapers	Resistance training	Crumbling provides good visual and tactile stimulation.	Crumble for hand strength. After crumbling, participants can throw the paper in a basket in front of them as a coordination and ROM activity. The ink tends to rub off on hands when crumbling. Some participants may dislike getting their hands dirty.
Paper plates	Resistance training	Arthritis	Create gentle air resistance by holding them during exercises.
Parachutes	ROM	Some parachutes have handles, and others do not. Be aware of participants who have limited ROM or who cannot hold onto the parachute for long.	Use for group and team play.
Pinwheels	Breathing exercises Relaxation	Multisensory tools that are helpful for those with COPD or with dementia or vision loss.	Useful for breathing exercises and for visual stimulation.
Plastic water bottles (20 ounces [591 milliliters] or less), filled with water, pennies, or sand.	Resistance training	Frail participants should start with 0.5-pound (0.2-kilogram) weights.	If the water bottles are sealed, drink the water after resistance training.
Puttylike substances	Resistance training	For participants who have arthritis in hands or hemiparesis or hemiplegia from a stroke.	Good for hand contractures and hand exercises.
Resistance bands and tubes	Resistance training Stretching	Ideal for participants at risk of dropping hand weights. Bands or tubes with handles can be easier to hold for individuals with arthritis in their hands or hemiparesis or hemiplegia from a stroke. Avoid placing bands or tubes around the legs and feet of diabetics, especially those with neuropathy.	Store in a dark, dry, cool place. Inspect them before using for holes or tears; discard damaged ones. Sharp objects (e.g., long fingernails and rings) can damage bands. Use firmer bands or tubes as a stretching prop. You can make handles with a loop and a knot in longer bands and tubes. For more information, see "Suggested Resources."

Type of equipment	Exercise component	Special needs/adaptations	How to use and other considerations
Ropes (soft)	Stretching	Helpful for those with limited ROM and flexibility.	Soft ropes can be used for upper- and lower-extremity exercises. Longer ropes work better for participants with limited ROM.
Socks, filled with beans or rice	Resistance training	For frail participants or those with dementia or arthritis in hands	Participants who are at risk of dropping hand weights can feel success by progressing from learning the resistance exercise with body weight to using hand weights in the form of filled socks.
Sponges (large and small)	Warm-ups Resistance training	Sponges have enough give to them that a frail participant can feel the effect of their motion on the sponge.	Large sponges can be squeezed between the knees as an isometric exercise, if this is safe for a participant. Smaller sponges can be used for hand and under-the-arm exercises.
Towels	Warm-ups Aerobics Resistance training Stretching	Helpful to extend the reach of those with limited ROM and flexibility. A folded towel can be placed under the feet of those whose legs do not touch the floor when seated.	Towels can be used for upper- and lower-extremity exercises. Longer towels work better for participants with limited ROM. Shorter towels are better for hand exercises.

A cart with wheels is recommended for storing and transporting exercise supplies.

MUSCLES OF THE HUMAN BODY

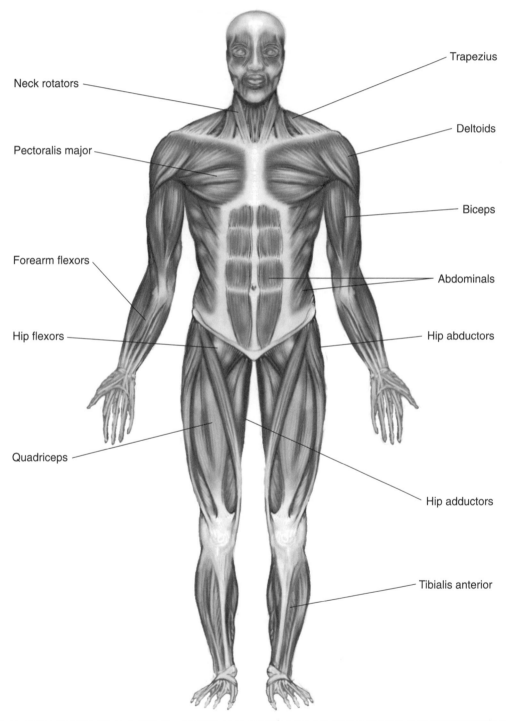

Neck rotators

Trapezius

Pectoralis major

Deltoids

Biceps

Forearm flexors

Abdominals

Hip flexors

Hip abductors

Quadriceps

Hip adductors

Tibialis anterior

Reprinted, by permission, from W.L. Westcott, 1999, *Strength training for seniors* (Champaign, IL: Human Kinetics), 42-43. From *Exercise for Frail Elders* by E. Best-Martini and K. A. Botenhagen-DiGenova, 2003, Champaign, IL: Human Kinetics.

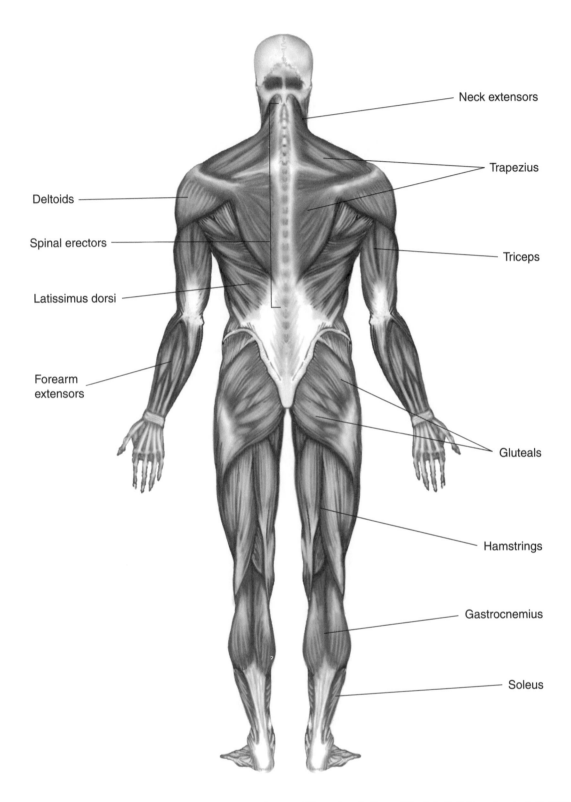

Neck extensors

Trapezius

Deltoids

Spinal erectors

Latissimus dorsi

Triceps

Forearm
extensors

Gluteals

Hamstrings

Gastrocnemius

Soleus

Reprinted, by permission, from W.L. Westcott, 1999, *Strength training for seniors* (Champaign, IL: Human Kinetics), 42-43. From *Exercise for Frail Elders* by E. Best-Martini and K. A. Botenhagen-DiGenova, 2003, Champaign, IL: Human Kinetics.

Resistance Training Log

Resistance training program of _____

(Name)

- The eight exercises marked by an asterisk are recommended for a shorter program.
- Use blank spaces for writing in alternative exercises or variations.
- Perform resistance exercises sitting upright, not leaning against the back of the chair, to strengthen torso (postural) muscles.
- Remember to stretch after your resistance training. Happy exercising!

Basic Seated Exercises or Standing Resistance Exercises		Date		Date		Date		Date		Date		Date		Date		Date		Date		Date	
Body region	**Exercise**	W	R	W	R	W	R	W	R	W	R	W	R	W	R	W	R	W	R	W	R
Chest Arms Shoulders	*6.1 Chest Press																				
Back Arms Shoulders	*6.2 Two-Arm Row																				
Shoulders Arms	*6.3 Overhead Press																				
Upper arms	6.4 Biceps Curl																				
	6.5 Triceps Extension (challenger)																				
Hip	*6.6 Modified Chair Stands (challenger)																				
Upper leg	*6.7 Hip Flexion																				
	*6.8 Hip Abduction and Adduction																				
	6.9 Knee Flexion																				
	6.10 Knee Extension																				
Lower leg	*6.11 Toe Raises																				
	*6.12 Heel Raises																				

W = weight; R = repetitions.

From *Exercise for Frail Elders* by E. Best-Martini and K. A. Botenhagen-DiGenova, 2003, Champaign, IL: Human Kinetics.

REFERENCES

Aaberg, E. 1998. *Muscle mechanics*. Champaign, IL: Human Kinetics.

American Association of Cardiovascular and Pulmonary Rehabilitation (AACVPR). 1998. *Guidelines for pulmonary rehabilitation programs*, 2nd ed. Champaign, IL: Human Kinetics.

———. 1999. *Guidelines for cardiac rehabilitation and secondary prevention programs*, 3rd ed. Champaign, IL: Human Kinetics.

American Association of Retired Persons, American College of Sports Medicine, American Geriatrics Society, Centers for Disease Control and Prevention, National Institute on Aging, and The Robert Wood Johnson Foundation. 2001. *National blueprint: Increasing physical activity among adults age 50 and older*. Available online: www.health.gov/healthypeople/document/pdf/uih/2010uih.pdf. (Accessed September 4, 2002.) Also available in *Journal of Aging and Physical Activity* 9 (Suppl).

American College of Sports Medicine (ACSM). 1994. Exercise for patients with coronary artery disease: Position stand. *Medicine and Science in Sport and Exercise* 26 (3): i–v.

———. 1995. Osteoporosis and exercise: Position stand. *Medicine and Science in Sport and Exercise* 27 (4): i–vii.

———. 1997. *Exercise management for persons with chronic diseases and disabilities*. Champaign, IL: Human Kinetics.

———. 1998a. Exercise and physical activity for older adults: Position stand. *Medicine and Science in Sport and Exercise* 30 (6): 992–1008.

———. 1998b. The recommended quantity and quality of exercise for developing and maintaining cardiorespiratory and muscular fitness, and flexibility in healthy adults: Position stand. *Medicine and Science in Sport and Exercise* 30 (6): 975–991.

American Psychiatric Association. 2000. *Diagnostic and statistical manual of mental disorders* (DSM), 4th ed. Washington, DC: American Psychiatric Association.

American Red Cross. 2003. *First aid manual*. Boston, MA: Staywell.

American Senior Fitness Association (SFA). 2003a. *Long term care fitness leader training manual*. New Smyrna Beach, FL: American Senior Fitness Association.

———. 2003b. *Senior fitness instructor training manual*. New Smyrna Beach, FL: American Senior Fitness Association.

———. 2003c. *Special population imperatives for custom older adult training*. New Smyrna Beach, FL: American Senior Fitness Association.

Anderson, B. 2000. *Stretching*. Bolinas, CA: Shelter.

Annesi, J.J., and W. Zimmerman. 1997. Senior programming for adherence to routine exercise. *Senior Fitness Bulletin* 4 (3): 9–11.

Baechle, T.R., and R.W. Earle, eds. 2000. *Essentials of strength training and conditioning*, 2nd ed. Champaign, IL: Human Kinetics.

Balady, G.J., K.A. Berra, L.A. Golding, N.F. Gordon, D.A. Mahler, J.N. Myers, and L.M. Sheldahl. 2000. *ACSM's guidelines for exercise testing and prescription*, 6th ed. Baltimore: Lippincott Williams & Wilkins.

Bandy, W.D., and B. Sanders. 2001. *Therapeutic exercise: Techniques for intervention*. Baltimore: Lippincott Williams & Wilkins.

Best Martini, E., M.A. Weeks, and P. Wirth. 2003. *Long term care for activity professionals, recreational therapists and social service professionals*, 4th ed. Ravensdale, WA: Idyll Arbor.

Blair, S.N., A.L. Dunn, B.H. Marcus, R.A. Carpenter, and P. Jaret. 2001. *Active living every day*. Champaign, IL: Human Kinetics

Blieszner, R., and R.G. Adams. 1992. *Adult friendship*. Thousand Oaks, CA: Sage.

Booth, D.S. 1998. *Clinicians handbook of exercise programs and patient instruction*, 2nd ed. Paradise, CA: Paradise West Medical Graphics.

Borg, G.A.V. 1998. *Borg's perceived exertion and pain scales*. Champaign, IL: Human Kinetics.

Brooks, G.A., T.D. Fahey, and T.P. White. 1996. *Exercise physiology: Human bioenergetics and its applications*, 2nd ed. Mountain View, CA: Mayfield.

Brown-Watson, A.V. 1999. *Still kicking: Restorative groups for frail older adults*. Baltimore: Health Professionals.

Caldwell, J.R. 1996. Exercise in the elderly: An overview. In: *Exercise programming for older adults*, ed. J. Clark. New York: Haworth.

California Department of Health Services: Institute for Health and Aging. California Osteoporosis Prevention and Education Program. 1998. Sacramento: California Department of Health Services.

Chin A Paw, M.J.M, N. de Jong, M. Stevens, P. Bult, and E.G. Schouten. 2001. Development of an exercise program for the frail elderly. *Journal of Aging and Physical Activity* 9 (4): 452–465.

Christensen, A. 1999. *The American Yoga Association easy does it yoga.* New York: Simon & Schuster.

Clark, J. 1992. *Full life fitness: A complete exercise program for mature adults.* Champaign, IL: Human Kinetics.

———. 1998. Older adult exercise techniques. In: *Exercise for older adults,* ed. R.T. Cotton. Champaign, IL: Human Kinetics.

———. 2003. *Seniorcise: A simple guide to fitness for the elderly and disabled,* 2nd ed. New Smyrna Beach, FL: American Senior Fitness Association.

Coleman, K.J., H.R. Raynor, D.M. Mueller, F.J. Cerny, J.M. Dorn, and L.H. Epstein. 1999. Providing sedentary adults with choices for meeting their walking goals. *Preventive Medicine* 28 (May): 510–519.

Copeland, M.E. 1994. *The depression workbook.* Oakland, CA: New Harbinger.

Cotton, R.T., C.J. Ekeroth, and H. Yancy, eds. 1998. *Exercise for older adults: ACE's guide for fitness professionals.* Champaign, IL: Human Kinetics.

Cousins, S.O. 1998. *Exercise, aging, and health.* Philadelphia: Taylor & Francis.

Cravern, S. 1998. A medical jigsaw puzzle: Depression and dementia in older adults. Dimensions 5 (4): 1.

Cross, K.M., and T.W. Worrell. 1999. Effects of a static stretching program on the incidence of lower extremity musculotendinous strains. *Journal of Athletic Training* 34: 11–14.

DeBusk, R.F., U. Stenestrand, M. Sheehan, and W.L. Haskell. 1990. Training effects of long versus short bouts of exercise in healthy subjects. *American Journal of Cardiology* 65: 1010–1013.

Delavier, F. 2001. *Strength training anatomy.* Champaign, IL: Human Kinetics.

Diamond, J. 1996. *Exercises for airplanes (and other confined spaces).* New York: Excalibur.

Dunn, A.L., M.H. Trivedi, and H.A. O'Neal. 2001. Physical activity dose-response effects on outcomes of depression and anxiety. *Medicine and Science in Sports and Exercise* 33 (6): S587–S597.

Duthie, E.H., and P.R. Katz, eds. 1998. *Practice of geriatrics,* 3rd ed. Philadelphia: Saunders.

Earle, R.W., and T.R. Baechle. 2000. Resistance training and spotting techniques. In *Essentials of strength training and conditioning,* 2nd ed., ed. T.R. Baechle and R.W. Earle. Champaign, IL: Human Kinetics.

Edginton, C.R., S.D. Hudson, and P.M. Ford. 1999. *Leadership in recreation and leisure services organizations.* Champaign, IL: Sagamore.

Ehsani, A.A. 1987. Cardiovascular adaptations to endurance exercise training in ischemic heart disease. *Exercise and Sport Sciences Review* 15: 53-66.

Evans, W.J. 1999. Exercise training guidelines for the elderly. *Medicine and Science in Sports and Exercise* 31 (1):12–17.

Exercise for the 50+ adult. 1997. IDEA Resource Series. San Diego: IDEA.

Feigenbaum, M.S., and M.L. Pollock. 1999. Prescription of resistance training for health and disease. *Medicine and Science in Sports and Exercise* 31 (1): 38–45.

Franks, B.D., and E.T. Howley. 1998. *Fitness leader's handbook,* 2nd ed. Champaign, IL: Human Kinetics.

Galdwin, L.A. 1991. Stretching: A valuable component of functional mobility training in the elderly. *Activities, Adaptation and Aging* 20 (3): 37–47.

Gordon, N.F. 1993. *Stroke: Your complete exercise guide.* The Cooper Clinic and Research Institute Fitness Series. Champaign, IL: Human Kinetics.

Graves, J.E., and B.A. Franklin, eds. 2001. *Resistance training for health and rehabilitation.* Champaign, IL: Human Kinetics.

Hall, C.M., and L.T Brody. 1999. *Therapeutic exercise: Moving toward function.* Philadelphia: Lippincott Williams & Wilkins.

Haskell, W.L. 2001. What to look for in assessing responsiveness to exercise in a health context. *Medicine and Science in Sport and Exercise* 33 (6): S454–S458.

Health Care Financing Administration. 1999. *HCFA's quality indicators and new survey procedures.* State Operations Manual Provider Certification (Transmittal No. 10, July 1999). Washington, DC: Health Care Financing Administration.

Hyatt, G. 2001. *Exercise and diabetes: Exercise for populations with special medical concerns.* Tucson, AZ: Desert Southwest Fitness.

Hyatt, G, and K.P. Nelson. 2002. *Exercise and arthritis: Exercise for populations with special medical concerns.* Tucson, AZ: Desert Southwest Fitness.

Kaiser Permanente. 1994. *Healthwise handbook.* Boise, ID: Healthwise.

Katsinas, R.P. 1995. Excess disability. Presented at American Therapeutic Recreation Society Conference, Louisville, KY.

Kelley, D.E., and B.H. Goodpaster. 2001. Effects of exercise on glucose homeostasis in type 2 diabetes mellitus. *Medicine and Science in Sports and Exercise* 33 (6): S495–S501.

Kesaniemi, Y.A., E. Danforth, Jr., M.D. Jensen, P.G. Kopelman, P. Lefebvre, and B.A. Reeder. 2001. Dose-response issues concerning physical activity and health:

An evidence-based symposium. *Medicine and Science in Sports and Exercise* 33 (6): S351–S358.

Kouzes, J., and B. Posner. 1995. *The leadership challenge: How to keep getting extraordinary things done in organizations.* San Francisco: Jossey Bass.

Lorig, K., H. Holman, D. Sobel, D. Laurent, V. Gonzalez, and M. Minor. 2000. *Living a healthy life with chronic conditions: Self-management of heart disease, arthritis, diabetes, asthma, bronchitis, emphysema and others,* 2nd ed. Palo Alto, CA: Bull.

MacBeth, L. 2001. *Exercise and Parkinson's disease.* Tucson, AZ: Desert Southwest Fitness.

Mazzeo, R.S. 2001. Exercise prescription for the elderly: Current recommendations. *Sports Medicine* 31 (11): 809–818.

McArdle, W.D., F.I. Katch, and V.L. Katch. 2000. *Essentials of exercise physiology,* 2nd ed. Baltimore: Lippincott Williams & Wilkins.

McCartney, N. 1999. Acute responses to resistance training and safety. *Medicine and Science in Sports and Exercise* 31 (1): 31–37.

McKelvey, S. 2003. *Functional fitness for older adults training manual.* San Diego, CA: Aging and Independence Services.

National Institute on Aging. 2000. *Older Americans.* Washington, DC: United States Department of Health and Human Services.

National Institutes of Health, Arthritis and Musculoskeletal and Skin Disease. 2001. Washington, DC: National Institutes of Health.

National Institutes of Health. 1995. Physical activity and cardiovascular health. *NIH Consensus Statement Online* 13 (3): 1–33. Available: http://consensus.nih.gov/cons/101/101_statement.htm [August 6, 2002].

Nelson, M.E., and S. Wernick. 2000. *Strong women stay young,* rev. ed. New York: Bantam Books.

O'Connor, G.T., J.E. Buring, S. Yusuf, S.Z. Goldhaber, E.M. Olmstead, R.S. Paffenbarger, and C.H. Hennekens. 1989. An overview of randomized trials of rehabilitation with exercise after myocardial infarction. *Circulation* 80: 234-244.

Osness, W.H., ed. 1998. *Exercise and the older adult.* Dubuque, IA; Kendall/Hunt.

Pate, R.R., M. Pratt, S.N. Blair, W.L. Haskell, C.A. Macera, C. Bouchard, D. Buchner, W. Ettinger, G.W. Heath, A.L. King, A. Kriska, A.S. Leon, B.H. Marcus, J. Morris, R.S. Paffenbarger, K. Patrick, M.L. Pollock, J.M. Rip pe, J. Sallis, and J.H. Wilmore. 1995. Physical activity and public health: A recommendation from the Centers for Disease Control and Prevention and the American College of Sports Medicine. *Journal of the American Medical Association* 273: 402–407.

Picone, R.E. 2000. Improving functional flexibility. In *Maximize your training: Insights from leading strength and fitness professionals,* ed. M. Brzycki. Lincolnwood, IL: Masters Press.

Pollock, M.L., J.E. Graves, D.L. Swart, and D.T Lowenthal. 1994. Exercise training and prescription for the elderly. *Southern Medical Journal* 87 (5): S88–S95.

Pryse-Phillips, W. 1989. Infarction of the medulla and cervical cord after fitness exercises. *Stroke* 20: 292–294.

Rowe, R.L., and J.W. Kahn. 1998. *Successful aging.* New York: Dell.

Salthouse, T. 1990. *Theoretical perspectives on cognitive aging.* Hillsdale, NJ: Lawrence Erlbaum.

Scheller, M.D. 1993. *Growing older feeling better in body, mind and spirit.* Palo Alto, CA: Bull.

Shepard, R.J. 1997. *Aging, physical activity and health.* Champaign, IL: Human Kinetics.

Singh, N., K. Clements, and M. Fiatarone. 1997. A randomized controlled trial of progressive resistance training in depressed elders. *Journal of Gerontology* 52A (1): M27–M35.

Sullivan, D.H., P.T. Wall, J.R. Bariola, M.M. Bopp, and Y.M. Frost. 2001. Progressive resistance muscle strength training of hospitalized frail elderly. *American Journal of Physical Medicine and Rehabilitation* 80 (7): 503–509.

Swart, D.L., M.L. Pollock, and W.F. Brechue. 1996. Aerobic exercise for older participants. In *Exercise programming for older adults,* ed. J. Clark. New York: Haworth.

Thomas, W. 1996. *Life worth living: An introduction to the principles and practices of the Eden alternative.* New York: VanderWyk & Burnham.

———. 2000. *Healthy People 2010: Understanding and improving health,* 2nd ed. Washington, DC: U.S. Government Printing Office. Available online: www.health.gov/healthypeople/document/pdf/uih/2010uih.pdf (Accessed: September 4, 2002).

U.S. Department of Health and Human Services. 2002. *Physical activity and older adults: Benefits and strategies.* Agency for Healthcare Research and Quality and the Centers for Disease Control. Available: www.ahrq.gov/ppip/activity.htm [August 6, 2002].

U.S. Surgeon General. 1996. *Physical activity and health: A report of the Surgeon General.* Atlanta, GA: U.S. Department of Health and Human Services, Centers for Disease Control and Prevention, National Center for Chronic Disease Prevention and Health Promotion.

Vincent, K.R., and R.W. Braith. 2002. Resistance exercise and bone turnover in elderly men and women. *Medicine and Science in Sports and Exercise* 34 (1): 17–23.

Vitti, K.A., C.M. Bayles, W.J. Carender, J.M. Prendergast, and F.J. D'Amico. 1993. A low-level strength training exercise program for frail elderly adults living in an extended attention facility. *Aging, Clinical and Experimental Research* 5 (5): 363–369.

Wescott, W.L., and T.R. Baechle. 1999. *Strength training for seniors: An instructor guide for developing safe and effective programs.* Champaign, IL: Human Kinetics.

Williford, H.N., J.B. East, F.H. Smith, and L.A. Burry. 1986. Evaluation of warm-up for improvement in flexibility. *American Journal of Sports Medicine* 14:316–319.

World Health Organization. 1997. The Heidelberg guidelines for promoting physical activity among older persons. *Journal of Aging and Physical Activity* 5 (1): 2–8.

YMCA of the USA. 1994. *YMCA strength training.* Champaign, IL: Human Kinetics.

———. 2000. *YMCA personal training instructor manual.* Champaign, IL: Human Kinetics.

Suggested Resources

Note: Refer to the References for additional resources.

Books and Manuals

Fitness, Health, and Special Needs

American College of Sports Medicine. 1997. *Exercise management for persons with chronic diseases and disabilities.* Champaign, IL: Human Kinetics.

Bond-Howard, B. 1993. *Introduction to stroke.* Ravensdale, WA: Idyll Arbor.

Bowlby, C. 1993. *Therapeutic activities with persons disabled by Alzheimer's disease and related disorders.* Gaithersburg, MD: Aspen.

Brown, A. 1999. *Still kicking: Restorative groups for frail older adults.* Baltimore: Health Professions.

Clark, J. 2003. *Seniorcise: A simple guide to fitness for the elderly and disabled,* 2nd ed. New Smyrna Beach, FL: American Senior Fitness Association.

Donatelle, R.J., and L.G. Davis. 1998. *Access to health.* Needham Heights, MA: Allyn & Bacon.

Hellen, C.R. 1998. *Alzheimer's disease: Activity-focused care.* Boston: Butterworth Heinemann.

Hurley, O. 1988. *Safe therapeutic exercise for the frail elderly: an introduction,* 2nd ed. Boston: MA.: The Center for the Study of Aging.

IDEA Resource Series. 1997. *Exercise for the 50+ adult.* San Diego, CA: IDEA.

National Institutes of Health, and the National Institute on Aging. 2001. *Exercise: A guide from the National Institute on Aging.* Bethesda, MD: National Institutes of Health/National Institute on Aging. Free publication. 800-222-2225.

Perkins-Carpenter, B. 1999. *How to prevent falls: A comprehensive guide to better balance.* Penfield, NY: Senior Fitness Productions.

Rikli, R.E., and C. Jessie Jones. 2001. *Senior fitness test manual.* Champaign, IL: Human Kinetics.

Sharkey, B.J. 2002. *Fitness and health,* 5th ed. Champaign, IL: Human Kinetics.

Winter Park Health Foundation. 1998. *Chairful wellness: A chairful method of helping older adults keep fit.* Winter Park, FL: Winter Park Health Foundation.

Inspirational

Clark, E. 1995. *Growing old is not for sissies II: Portraits of senior athletes.* San Francisco: Pomegranate Artbooks.

Ferrin, K. 1999. *What's age got to do with it? Secret to aging in extraordinary ways.* San Diego: ALTI. 800-284-8537.

Rowe, J.W., and R.L. Kahn. 1998. *Successful aging.* New York: Dell.

Relaxation and Stress Reduction

Dworkis, S. 1997. *Recovery yoga: A practical guide for chronically ill, injured, and post-operative people.* New York: Three Rivers.

Kabat-Zinn, J. 1990. *Full catastrophe living (program of the Stress Reduction Clinic at University of Massachusetts Medical Center).* New York: Dell.

Korb-Khalsa, K.L., and E.A Leutenberg. 2000. *Life management skills VII.* Beachwood, OH: Wellness Reproductions.

Scheller, M.D. 1993. *Growing older feeling better in body, mind and spirit.* Palo Alto, CA: Bull.

Reference

Berkow, R., M.H. Beers, R.M. Bogin, and A.J. Fletcher, eds. 2000. *Merck manual of medical information.* New York: Simon & Schuster.

Dirckx, J.H., ed. 2001. *Stedman's concise medical dictionary for the health professions*, illus. 4th ed. Baltimore: Lippincott Williams & Wilkins.

Kapit, W., and L.M. Elson. 1993. *The anatomy coloring book*, 2nd ed. Reading, MA: Addison-Wesley.

Seig, K.W., and S.P. Adams. 2002. *Illustrated essentials of musculoskeletal anatomy*, 4th ed. Gainesville, FL: Megabooks.

RESISTANCE BANDS AND TUBES

Corning Creager, C. 1998. Therapeutic exercises using resistive bands. Berthoud, CO: Executive Physical Therapy. 800-367-7393.

Schleck, L.A., ed. 2000. Staying strong: A senior's guide to a more active and independent life. Minneapolis, MN: Fairview Press. 800-544-8207.

CONTINUING EDUCATION

American Senior Fitness Association. 2003. *Long term care fitness leader training manual*. New Smyrna Beach, FL: American Senior Fitness Association. 800-243-1478.

———. 2003. *Senior fitness instructor training manual*. New Smyrna Beach, FL: American Senior Fitness Association.

———. 2003. *Senior personal trainer training manual*. New Smyrna Beach, FL: American Senior Fitness Association.

Bovre, S. 2001. *Balance training: A program for improving balance in older adults*. Tucson, AZ: Desert Southwest Fitness. 800-873-6759.

Hyatt, G. 1998. *Exercise and urinary incontinence*. Tucson, AZ: Desert Southwest Fitness. 800-873-6759.

CERTIFICATIONS

Long Term Care Fitness Leader; Senior Personal Trainer; Senior Fitness Instructor
American Senior Fitness Association
P.O. Box 2575
New Smyrna Beach, FL 32170
800-243-1478

Exercise for Adults With Special Needs Instructor Certification
College of Marin
835 College Avenue
Kentfield, CA 94904
415-453-6130

JOURNALS AND NEWSLETTERS

Creative Forecasting. A monthly newsletter for activity and recreation professionals. P.O. Box 7789, Colorado Springs, CO 80937-7789. 719-633-3174. cfi@cfactive.com.

Journal of Aging and Physical Activity. Champaign, IL: Human Kinetics. 800-747-4457. www.HumanKinetics.com.

VIDEOS

Alan, K. 1997. Age is the rage! Part 2: Seated and standing aerobics. Los Angeles: Ken Alan Associates. 323-653-5040.

Gladwin, L.A. 2000. Movin' out senior style, phases I and II: Seated and standing aerobics, 2nd ed. New Smyrna Beach, FL: American Senior Fitness Association. 386-423-6634.

Knopf, K.G. 1999. Feeling fit & over sixty. Fitness Educators Of Older Adults Association, 759 Chopin Drive, Ste. 1, Sunnyvale CA 94087. 408-450-1224.

Marin County Division on Aging. 1998. Strength training for older adults. Marin County Division on Aging, 10 North San Pedro Road, Suite 1012, San Rafael, CA 94903. 415-499-7396.

Murphy, J.M. 2002. Conscious aging with yoga: Volume 1. Beginning in a chair. Sausalito, CA: Integrated Resources. 415-339-8879.

———. 2003. Conscious aging with yoga: Volume 2. Transitioning to standing. Sausalito, CA: Integrated Resources. 415-339-8879.

Stolove, J. 1996. Chair dancing: A new concept in aerobics fitness. Del Mar, CA: Chair Dancing International. 800-551-4386. www.chairdancing.com.

———. 1996. Chair dancing around the world. Del Mar, CA: Chair Dancing International.

———. 2002. Chair dancing through the decades—moves and music for the best of times. Del Mar, CA: Chair Dancing International.

Tahoe Forest Hospital. 1998. Fitness forever: The exercise program for healthy aging! Champaign, IL: Human Kinetics.

Wilson, M.A. 1995. Sit and be fit: All sitting exercises. Spokane, WA: Sit and Be Fit. 509-448-9438. www.sitandbefit.com.

———. 1995. Sit and be fit: Caregivers guide to exercise. Spokane, WA: Sit and Be Fit.

———. 1995. Sit and be fit: Tone and stretch IV. Spokane, WA: Sit and Be Fit.

———. 2000. Sit and be fit: All American workout. Spokane, WA: Sit and Be Fit.

RELAXATION AND STRESS REDUCTION TAPES

Emmett. E. Miller, MD
P.O. Box W
Stanford, CA 94309
800-528-2737

Mindfulness Meditation Tapes
Stress Reduction Tapes
Jon Kabat-Zinn, PhD
P.O. Box 547
Lexington, MA 02420

Center for Mindfulness
UMass Medical Center
Shaw Bldg., 55 Lake Ave. North
Worcester, MA 01605
508-856-2000
www.umassmed.edu/cfm

Exercise Sources

Briggs. 800-247-2343. www.BriggsCorp.com

Flaghouse. 800-265-6900. www.flaghouse.com

Nasco. 800-558-9595. www.eNASCO.com

Seabay. 800-568-0188. www.seabaygame.com

S&S Primelife. 800-243-9232. www.ssww.com

Music Sources

Ken Alan Associates. 323-653-5040.

Musicflex. 718-738-6839.

Power Productions. 800-777-2328.

Sports Music, Inc. 800-878-4764.

Professional Organizations and Foundations

Aerobics and Fitness Association of America
15250 Ventura Blvd., Ste. 200
Sherman Oaks, CA 91403-3297
800-446-2322
www.afaa.com

Alliance for Aging Research
2021 K Street, NW, Ste. 305
Washington, DC 20006
202-293-2856
www.agingresearch.org

American Alliance for Health, Physical Education, Recreation and Dance (AAHPERD)
1900 Association Dr.
Arlington, VA 20191-1598
800-213-7193
www.aahperd.org

American Association of Retired Persons (AARP)
601 E St., NW
Washington, DC 20049
800-424-3410
www.aarp.org

American College of Sports Medicine (ACSM)
401 W. Michigan St.
Indianapolis, IN 46202-3233
800-486-5643
www.acsm.org

American Council on Exercise (ACE)
4851 Paramount Dr.
San Diego, CA 92123
800-825-3636
www.acefitness.com

American Diabetes Association
1701 Beauregard St.
Alexandria, VA 22311
800-342-2383
www.diabetes.org

American Health Care Association
1201 L St., NW
Washington, DC 20005
202-842-4444
www.ahca.org

American Heart Association
7272 Greenville Ave.
Dallas, TX 75231
800-242-8721
www.americanheart.org

American Lung Association
61 Broadway, 6th Floor
New York, NY 10006
800-586-4872
www.lungusa.org

American Parkinson Disease Association, Inc.
1250 Hylan Blvd., Ste. 4B
Staten Island, NY 10305-1946
800-223-2732
www.apdaparkinson.org

American Senior Fitness Association (SFA)
P.O. Box 2575
New Smyrna Beach, FL 32170
800-243-1478
www.seniorfitness.net

American Society on Aging
833 Market St., Ste. 511
San Francisco, CA 94103-1824
800-537-9728
www.asaging.org

American Therapeutic Recreation Association
1414 Prince St., Ste. 104
Alexandria, VA 22314
703-683-9420
www.atra-tr.org

Arthritis Foundation
P.O. Box 7669
Atlanta, GA 30357-0669
800-283-7800
www.arthritis.org

Cooper Institute for Aerobics Research
12330 Preston Rd.
Dallas, TX 75230
800-635-7050
www.cooperinst.org

Desert Southwest Fitness, Inc.
Center for Continuing Education
602 E. Roger Rd.
Tucson, AZ 85705
800-873-6759
www.dswfitness.com

50-Plusfitness Association
1040 Noel Dr., Ste. 100
Menlo Park, CA 94025
650-323-6160
www.50plus.org

Fitness Educators of Older Adults Association
759 Chopin Drive, Ste. 1
Sunnyvale, CA 94087
408-450-1244
www.fitnesseducators.com

International Dance Exercise Association (IDEA)
6190 Cornerstone Ct. E., Ste. 204
San Diego, CA 92121-3773
800-999-4332, ext. 7
www.ideafit.com

International Society for Aging and Physical Activity
    (ISAPA)
Wojtek Chodzko-Zajko, PhD
University of Illinois Department of Kinesiology
Louise Freer Hall, 906 S. Goodwin Ave.
Urbana, IL 61801
217-244-0823
www.isapa.org

Keiser Institute on Aging
Keiser Corporation
2470 Cherry Ave.
Fresno, CA 93706
800-888-7009
www.keiserinstituteonaging.com

National Academy on an Aging Society
1030 15th St., NW, Ste. 250
Washington, DC 20005
202-842-1275
www.agingsociety.org

National Alzheimer's Association
919 N. Michigan Ave., Ste. 1100
Chicago, IL 60611-1676
800-272-3900
www.alz.org

National Association of Activity Professionals
P.O. Box 5530
Sevierville, TN 37866
865-429-0717
www.thenaap.com

National Council on Assisted Living
1201 L St., NW
Washington, DC 20005
202-842-4444
www.ncal.org

National Institute on Aging
Building 31, Room 5C27
31 Center Dr., MSC 2292
Bethesda, MD 20892
800-222-2225
www.nia.nih.gov

National Recreation and Parks Association
22377 Belmont Ridge Rd.
Ashburn, VA 20148-4501
703-858-0784
www.nrpa.org

National Strength and Conditioning Association
NSCA Certification Committee
1640 L St., Ste. G
Lincoln, NE 68508
888-746-2378
www.nsca-cc.org

National Therapeutic Recreation Society (NTRS)
NRPA, 22377 Belmont Ridge Rd.
Ashburn, VA 20148-4501
703-858-0784
703-858-0174
www.nrpa.org

SeniorAct—Activities for a Geriatric Setting
www.senioract.com

U.S. Office of Disease Prevention and Health Promotion,
    Healthy People 2010
U.S. Government Printing Office
710 N. Capitol St., NW
Washington, DC 20401
202-512-0132
www.health.gov/healthypeople

PROFESSIONAL LIABILITY INSURANCE

International Dance Exercise Association (IDEA). 800-
    999-4332, ext. 7. www.ideafit.com/insurance.htm

INDEX

Page numbers followed by *f* or *t* indicate pages with figures and tables.

ABOUT THE AUTHORS

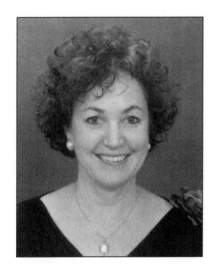

Elizabeth (Betsy) Best-Martini, MS, is a certified recreation therapist specializing in the field of gerontology and long-term care. She received her master's degree in recreation therapy and is a consultant to various retirement communities, skilled nursing settings, subacute settings, and residential and assisted care facilities in northern California. In addition to running her consulting firm, she lectures and provides training across the United States and in Canada. Two of her publications—*Long Term Care* and *Quality Assurance for Activity Programs*—are used nationally as textbooks.

Betsy is also an instructor at College of Marin and Santa Rosa Junior College, where she trains people to work with elderly clients as activity coordinators. In addition, she teaches two living history classes for older adults and a strength training class for frail elderly clients. Betsy is a certified long-term care fitness leader through the American Senior Fitness Association and a qualified strength trainer through the YMCA.

Betsy writes a column titled "Let's Get Moving" in *Creative Forecasting*, a national newsletter for activity professionals and recreation therapists. This column focuses on fitness programs for older adults. She has been recognized with the 1998 Distinguished Merit Award from NCCAC (Northern California Council of Activity Coordinators) and the Pete Croughan Award for her volunteer efforts with a nonprofit organization called LITA (Love Is The Answer).

In her leisure time, Betsy can be found gardening, hiking, exercising, and spending time with her husband and family.

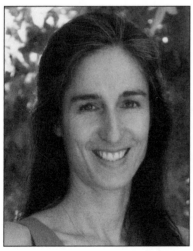

Kim A. Botenhagen-DiGenova, MA, received her master's degree in physical education (exercise physiology) and the Distinguished Achievement in a Major Field Award from San Francisco State University. She is certified by the American College of Sports Medicine as a health and fitness instructor; by the American Senior Fitness Association as a long-term care fitness leader, senior fitness leader, and senior personal trainer; and by the YMCA as a strength training instructor trainer. She is also a certified emergency medical technician and nutrition assistant.

Kim was the first exercise physiologist at the Davies Medical Center Health Check Department in San Francisco, where she worked for seven years. She now teaches Strength and Fitness Training for Older Adults and Exercise for Adults With Special Needs Instructor Certification Course at the College of Marin. She is the Northern California tester for the Amerian Senior Fitness Association and a consultant and workshop leader on fitness for older adults.

Kim lives in Novato, California. Her passions are swimming in San Francisco Bay and hiking. She has swum from the Golden Gate Bridge to the San Francisco-Oakland Bay Bridge and has successfully escaped from Alcatraz many times.

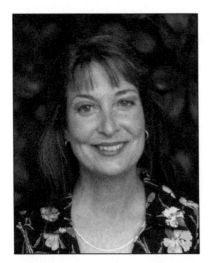

Janie Clark, MA, is president of the American Senior Fitness Association (SFA), the international organization for fitness professionals who serve older adults. Her master's degree from the University of Central Florida is in exercise physiology and wellness management. She is the author of numerous books including *Seniorcise: a Simple Guide to Fitness for the Elderly and Disabled; Full Life Fitness: A Complete Exercise Program for Mature Adults;* and *Exercise Programming for Older Adults* (Haworth Press). She has authored hundreds of articles for periodicals including the *Journal of Aging and Physical Activity; Activity, Adaptation & Aging Journal; ACE Certified News;* and *Modern Maturity.* She also served as a reviewer for the Rikli/Jones LifeSpan project that developed functional fitness tests for older adults and as a member of the Coalition to Develop National Curriculum Standards for Senior Fitness Professionals.

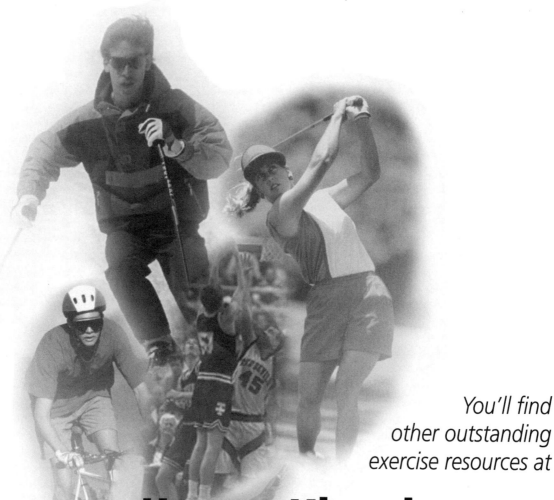

You'll find
other outstanding
exercise resources at

www.HumanKinetics.com

In the U.S. call

1-800-747-4457

Australia.. 08 8277 1555
Canada 1-800-465-7301
Europe... +44 (0) 113 255 5665
New Zealand....................................... 0064 9 448 1207

 HUMAN KINETICS
The Information Leader in Physical Activity
P.O. Box 5076 • Champaign, IL 61825-5076 USA